*Quick*FACTS™

Melanoma
SKIN CANCER

*Quick*FACTS™

From the Experts at the American Cancer Society

Melanoma
SKIN CANCER

What You Need to Know—NOW

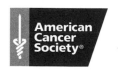

Published by the American Cancer Society/Health Promotions
250 Williams Street NW, Atlanta, Georgia 30303 USA

Copyright ©2012 American Cancer Society

Printed in the United States of America
Cover designed by Jill Dible, Atlanta, GA
Composition by Graphic Composition, Inc.

5 4 3 2 1   12 13 14 15 16

Library of Congress Cataloging-in-Publication Data

Melanoma skin cancer : what you need to know—now / from
the experts at the American Cancer Society.
     p. cm. — (Quickfacts)
  Includes bibliographical references and index.
  ISBN 978-1-60443-038-7 (pbk. : alk. paper)
  ISBN 1-60443-038-9 (pbk. : alk. paper)
  1. Melanoma—Popular works. 2. Skin—Cancer—
Popular works. I. American Cancer Society.
RC280.M37M47 2012
616.99'477—dc22

                   2011012075

Quantity discounts on bulk purchases of this book are
available. Book excerpts can also be created to fit specific
needs. For information, please contact the American Cancer
Society, Health Promotions Publishing, 250 Williams Street
NW, Atlanta, GA 30303-1002, or send an e-mail to
trade.sales@cancer.org.

A Note to the Reader

This information represents the views of the doctors and nurses serving on the American Cancer Society's Cancer Information Database Editorial Board. These views are based on their interpretation of studies published in medical journals, as well as their own professional experience.

The treatment information in this book is not official policy of the Society and is not intended as medical advice to replace the expertise and judgment of your cancer care team. It is intended to help you and your family make informed decisions, together with your doctor.

Your doctor may have reasons for suggesting a treatment plan different from these general treatment options. Don't hesitate to ask him or her questions about your treatment options.

For more information, contact your American Cancer Society at **800-227-2345** or **cancer.org**.

TABLE OF CONTENTS

Questions to Ask

After Treatment

Latest Research

Resources

Your Melanoma Skin Cancer

What Is Cancer?

The body is made up of hundreds of millions of living cells. Normal body cells grow, divide, and die in an orderly fashion. During the early years of a person's life, normal cells divide faster to allow the person to grow. After the person becomes an adult, most cells divide only to replace worn-out or dying cells or to repair injuries.

Cancer* begins when **cells** in a part of the body start to grow out of control. There are many kinds of cancer, but they all start because of out-of-control growth of abnormal cells. Cancer cell growth is different from normal cell growth. Instead of dying, cancer cells continue to grow and form new, abnormal cells. **Cancer cells** can also invade (grow into) other **tissues**, something that normal cells cannot do. Growing out of control and

---

*Terms in **bold type** are further explained in the glossary, beginning on page 119.

invading other tissues are what makes a cell a cancer cell.

Cells become cancer cells because of damage to **DNA**. DNA is in every cell and directs all its actions. In a normal cell, when DNA is damaged, the cell either repairs the damage or the cell dies. In cancer cells, the damaged DNA is not repaired, but the cell does not die like it should. Instead, this cell goes on making new cells that the body does not need. These new cells will all have the same damaged DNA as the first cell.

People can inherit damaged DNA, but most DNA damage is caused by mistakes that happen while the normal cell is reproducing or by something in the environment. Sometimes the cause of the DNA damage is something obvious, like cigarette smoking. Often, however, no clear cause is found.

In most cases, the cancer cells form a **tumor**. Some cancers, such as leukemia, rarely form tumors. Instead, these cancer cells involve the blood and blood-forming organs and circulate through other tissues where they grow.

Cancer cells often travel to other parts of the body, where they begin to grow and form new tumors that replace normal tissue. This process is called **metastasis**. It happens when the cancer cells get into the bloodstream or lymph vessels of the body.

No matter where a cancer may **metastasize**, or spread, it is always named for the place where it started. For example, breast cancer that has spread to the liver is still called breast cancer, not liver cancer.

Likewise, prostate cancer that has spread to the bone is **metastatic** prostate cancer, not bone cancer.

Different types of cancer can behave very differently. For example, lung cancer and breast cancer are very different diseases. They grow at different rates and respond to different treatments. That is why people with cancer need treatment that is aimed at their particular kind of cancer.

Not all tumors are **malignant**. Tumors that are not cancer are called **benign**. Benign tumors can cause problems—they can grow very large and press on healthy organs and tissues. However, they cannot invade other tissues. Because they cannot invade other tissues, they also cannot metastasize, or spread, to other parts of the body. These tumors are almost never life threatening.

What Is Melanoma?

Melanoma is a cancer that starts in a certain type of skin cell. To understand melanoma, it helps to know about the normal structure and function of the skin.

Normal Skin

Skin is the largest organ in your body. It does several different things:

- covers the internal organs and protects them from injury
- serves as a barrier to germs such as bacteria
- prevents the loss of too much water and other fluids
- helps control body temperature

The skin has the following 3 layers:
- epidermis
- dermis
- subcutis

Epidermis

The top layer of skin is the **epidermis**. The epidermis is very thin, averaging only 0.2 millimeters (mm) thick (about 1/100 of an inch). It protects the deeper layers of skin and the organs of the body from the environment.

Keratinocytes are the main cell type of the epidermis. These cells make an important protein called **keratin**, which gives the skin strength and flexibility and makes the skin waterproof.

The epidermis itself is made up of 3 sublayers. The outermost part of the epidermis is called the **stratum corneum**, or horny layer. It is composed of dead keratinocytes that are continually shed as new cells form. The cells in this layer are called **squamous cells** because of their flat shape.

Just below the stratum corneum are living keratinocytes. Below that is the basal layer, the inner

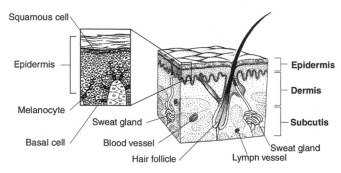

Squamous cell

Epidermis

Melanocyte

Basal cell

Sweat gland

Blood vessel

Hair follicle

Epidermis

Dermis

Subcutis

Sweat gland

Lymph vessel

layer of the epidermis. The cells of the basal layer, called **basal cells**, continually divide to form new keratinocytes. These new keratinocytes replace the older keratinocytes that slough off the skin's surface.

Melanocytes, the cells that can become melanoma, are also present in the epidermis. These skin cells make the brown pigment called **melanin**, which makes skin tan or brown. Melanin protects the deeper layers of the skin from some of the harmful effects of the sun.

The epidermis is separated from the deeper layers of skin by the **basement membrane**. The basement membrane is an important structure. When a cancer becomes more advanced, it generally grows through the basement membrane.

Dermis

The middle layer of the skin is called the **dermis**. The dermis is much thicker than the epidermis. It contains hair follicles, sweat glands, blood vessels, and nerves that are held in place by a protein called **collagen**. Collagen is made by cells called **fibroblasts** and gives the skin its resilience and strength.

Subcutis

The deepest layer of the skin is called the **subcutis**. The subcutis and the lowest part of the dermis form a network of collagen and fat cells. The subcutis helps the body conserve heat and has a shock-absorbing effect that helps protect the body's organs from injury.

Benign Skin Tumors

Many types of benign (noncancerous) tumors can develop from different types of skin cells.

Melanocytic tumors

A **mole**, or **nevus**, is a benign skin tumor that develops from melanocytes. Nearly all moles are harmless, but having some types may raise your risk of melanoma. See the section "What Are The Risk Factors for Melanoma?" on page 11 for more information about moles.

A **Spitz nevus** is a kind of skin tumor that sometimes looks like melanoma. These tumors are generally benign and do not spread. However, sometimes doctors have trouble telling Spitz nevi from true melanomas, even when looking at them under a microscope. Therefore, they are often removed, just to be safe.

Other benign tumors

Benign tumors that develop from other types of skin cells include the following:

- **seborrheic keratoses:** tan, brown, or black raised spots with a "waxy" texture or rough surface
- **hemangiomas:** benign blood vessel growths often called cherry or strawberry spots or port wine stains
- **lipomas:** soft growths of benign fat cells
- **warts:** rough-surfaced growths caused by a virus

Most of these tumors rarely, if ever, develop into cancers. There are a lot of other kinds of benign skin tumors, but most are not very common.

Melanoma

Melanoma is a cancer that begins in the melanocytes. Other names for this cancer include malignant melanoma and cutaneous melanoma. Because most melanoma cells still produce melanin, melanoma tumors are usually brown or black. This is not always true, however, as melanomas can be non-pigmented (without color).

Melanomas can occur anywhere on the skin but are more likely to start in certain locations. The trunk (chest and back) is the most common site in men. The legs are the most commonly affected site in women. The neck and face are other common sites for both men and women.

Having darkly pigmented skin lowers your risk, but it is not a guarantee—anyone can get melanoma. Melanoma can develop on the palms of the hands, the soles of the feet, and under the nails. Melanomas in these areas represent more than half of all melanomas in blacks but fewer than 10% of melanomas in whites.

Melanomas can form in other parts of the body such as the eyes, mouth, and vagina, but melanomas in these locations are much less common than melanoma of the skin. For more information about melanomas in these organs, contact the American Cancer Society at **800-227-2345**, or visit our Web site, **cancer.org**.

Melanoma is much less common than basal cell and squamous cell skin cancers (discussed below), but it is far more dangerous. Like basal cell and squamous cell skin cancers, melanoma is almost always curable in its early stages. However, it is much more likely than basal or squamous cell cancers to spread to other parts of the body if not caught early.

Other Skin Cancers

Skin cancers that are not melanoma are sometimes grouped together as **nonmelanoma skin cancers** because they develop from skin cells other than melanocytes. They tend to behave very differently from melanomas and are often treated in different ways.

Nonmelanoma skin cancers include **basal cell cancer** and **squamous cell cancer.** Basal cell and squamous cell skin cancers are by far the most common skin cancers and are actually more common than any other form of cancer. Because they rarely metastasize (spread elsewhere in the body), basal cell and squamous cell skin cancers are less worrisome and are treated differently from melanomas. **Merkel cell carcinoma** is an uncommon type of skin cancer that is sometimes harder to treat.

For information about these and other types of nonmelanoma skin cancers, contact your American Cancer Society at **800-227-2345** and request the documents *Skin Cancer—Basal and Squamous Cell, Kaposi Sarcoma, or Lymphoma of the Skin,* or visit our Web site, **cancer.org**. Basal and squamous cell skin cancers are also discussed in the American Cancer Society book *QuickFACTS™ Basal and Squamous Cell Skin Cancer.*

What Are the Key Statistics About Melanoma?

Skin cancer is by far the most common of all cancers. Melanoma accounts for less than 5% of skin cancer cases but causes most skin cancer deaths.

The American Cancer Society estimates that about 70,230 new melanomas will be diagnosed in the United States during 2011 (about 40,010 in men; 30,220 in women). Incidence rates for melanoma have been increasing for at least 30 years. In recent years, the increases have been most pronounced in young white women and in older white men.

Melanoma is more than 10 times more common in whites than in blacks. It is slightly more common in men than in women. Overall, the lifetime risk of melanoma is about 2% (1 in 50) for whites, 0.1% (1 in 1,000) for blacks, and 0.5% (1 in 200) for Hispanics. The risk for each person can be affected by a number of different factors, which are described in the section "What Are the Risk Factors for Melanoma?"

Unlike many other common cancers, melanoma has a wide age distribution. It occurs in younger and older people. Rates increase with age and are highest among people in their 80s, but melanoma is not uncommon even among people younger than 30. It is one of the most common cancers in young adults.

About 8,790 people in the United States are expected to die of melanoma during 2011 (about 5,750 men and 3,040 women). The death rate has been dropping since the 1990s for people younger than 50 but has been stable or rising in people older than 50.

For information on survival rates for melanoma, see the section "How Is Melanoma Staged?"

Risk Factors and Causes

What Are the Risk Factors for Melanoma?

A **risk factor** is anything that affects your chance of having a disease such as cancer. Different types of cancer have different risk factors. For example, smoking is a risk factor for cancers of the lung, mouth, larynx (voice box), bladder, kidney, and several other organs.

Risk factors do not tell us everything, however. Having a risk factor, or even several risk factors, does not mean that you will get the disease. Melanoma develops in many people who do not have any known risk factors. Even if a person with melanoma has a risk factor, it can be difficult to know how much that risk factor may have contributed to the cancer.

Scientists have found several risk factors that may place you at higher risk for melanoma.

Exposure to Ultraviolet Radiation

Exposure to **ultraviolet (UV) radiation** is the main risk factor for most melanomas. Sunlight is the main source of UV radiation, which can damage the **genes** in your skin cells. Tanning lamps, beds, and booths are also sources of UV radiation. People with high levels of exposure to radiation from these sources are at greater risk for skin cancer, including melanoma.

Ultraviolet radiation is divided into 3 wavelength ranges:

- **UVA rays** cause cells to age and can cause some damage to cells' DNA. They are linked to long-term skin damage such as wrinkles, but they are also thought to play a role in some skin cancers.
- **UVB rays** can cause direct damage to the DNA, and they are the rays that primarily cause sunburns. They are also thought to cause most skin cancers.
- **UVC rays** do not penetrate our atmosphere. They are not a cause of skin cancer.

Although UVA and UVB rays make up only a very small portion of the sun's wavelengths, they are the main cause of the sun's damaging effects on the skin. UV radiation damages the DNA of skin cells. Skin cancers begin when this damage affects the DNA of genes that control skin cell growth. Both UVA and UVB rays damage skin and cause skin cancer. UVB rays are a more potent cause of at least some skin cancers, but based on what is known today, there are *no* safe UV rays.

The amount of exposure to UV radiation depends on the intensity of the radiation, the length of time the skin was exposed, and whether the skin was protected with clothing and sunscreen.

The nature of the UV exposure may play a role in melanoma development. Many studies have linked the development of melanoma on the legs, arms, and trunk of the body to frequent sunburns, especially in childhood. The fact that these areas are not constantly exposed to UV radiation may also be important. Some experts think that melanomas in these areas are different from melanomas on the face and neck, where sun exposure is more constant. Melanomas that develop on areas where there has been little or no sun exposure, such as the palms of the hands, soles of the feet, underneath the nails, or internal surfaces such as the mouth and vagina, are different from either of the other types of melanoma.

For information on how to protect yourself and your family from UV exposure, see the section "Can Melanoma Be Prevented?" on page 19.

Moles

A **nevus**, or mole, is a benign melanocytic tumor. Moles are not usually present at birth, but they begin to appear in childhood. Most moles will never cause any problems, but a person who has many moles is at higher risk for melanoma.

Dysplastic nevi

A **dysplastic nevus** may look a little like a normal mole and a little like melanoma. They are often larger than other moles and have an abnormal shape or color. (See the section "Can Melanoma Be Found Early?" on pages 27–28 for descriptions of the appearance of moles and melanomas.) Dysplastic nevi can appear in areas that are exposed to the sun and in areas that are usually covered, such as the buttocks and scalp.

A small number of dysplastic nevi develop into melanomas, but most dysplastic nevi never become cancerous. Many melanomas seem to arise without a preexisting dysplastic nevus.

Lifetime melanoma risk may be higher than 10% for those with many dysplastic nevi, a condition sometimes referred to as dysplastic nevus syndrome. Dysplastic nevi often run in families. Lifetime risk goes up if the person also has close relatives who have had melanoma. A person with a large number of dysplastic nevi and several close relatives who have had melanoma has a 50% or greater lifetime risk of melanoma.

People with dysplastic nevus syndrome should have periodic thorough skin examinations performed by a dermatologist (a doctor who specializes in skin problems). In some cases, full body photographs are taken to help the doctor recognize which moles are changing and growing. Many doctors recommend that people be taught to do monthly skin self-examinations and be counseled about sun protection.

Congenital melanocytic nevi

Moles present at birth are called **congenital melanocytic nevi**. The lifetime risk of melanoma developing for people with congenital melanocytic nevi has been estimated to be between 0% and 10%, depending on the size of the nevus. People with very large congenital nevi have a greater risk, while the risk is smaller for those with small nevi.

Congenital nevi are sometimes removed by surgery so that they do not have a chance to become cancerous. The decision to remove a congenital nevus is influenced by several factors, including its size, location, and color. Many doctors recommend that congenital nevi be examined regularly by a dermatologist. People with congenital nevi should also be taught how to do monthly skin self-examinations.

The chance of any single mole turning into cancer is very low. However, anyone with lots of irregular or large moles has an increased risk of melanoma.

Fair Skin, Freckling, and Light Hair

The risk of melanoma is more than 10 times higher for whites than for blacks. This is because skin pigment has a protective effect. Whites with red or blond hair or fair skin that freckles or burns easily are at increased risk. Red-haired people have the highest risk.

Family History of Melanoma

Your risk of melanoma is greater if one or more of your **first-degree relatives** (mother, father, brother, sister, or child) has had melanoma. Around 10% of all people with melanoma have a family history of the disease.

The increased risk might be due to a shared family lifestyle of frequent sun exposure, a family tendency toward fair skin, or a combination of both factors. It may also be caused by inherited gene changes, or **mutations**. Gene mutations have been found in anywhere from about 10% to 40% of families with a high rate of melanoma. At this time, most experts do not recommend genetic testing in families with increased risk. Rather, they advise that people with a strong family history of melanoma do the following:

- have regular skin examinations by a dermatologist
- thoroughly examine their skin once a month
- be particularly careful about sun protection and avoid tanning beds

Personal History of Melanoma

A person who has already had melanoma is at increased risk for another melanoma. About 5% to 10% of people who have had melanoma will develop a second one at some point.

Immune Suppression

People who have been treated with medicines that suppress the immune system, such as people who have undergone an organ transplant, are at increased risk for melanoma.

Age

Although melanoma is not as closely linked to aging as most other types of cancer, it is still more likely to occur in older people. However, it is also found in younger people. Melanoma is one of the most common cancers in people younger than 30. Melanoma that runs in families may occur at a younger age.

Gender

In the United States, men have a higher rate of melanoma than women.

Xeroderma Pigmentosum

Xeroderma pigmentosum (XP) is a rare inherited condition that reduces the skin's ability to repair damage to DNA caused by sun exposure. People with XP have a high risk of both melanoma and basal cell and squamous cell skin cancers, usually starting in childhood. Because people with XP are less able to repair DNA damage caused by UV exposure, they are at higher risk for multiple cancers to develop on sun-exposed areas of their skin.

Do We Know What Causes Melanoma?

Researchers are beginning to understand how certain changes in DNA can make normal cells become cancerous. DNA is the chemical in each of our cells that makes up our genes—the instructions for how our cells function. We usually look like our parents because they are the source of our DNA. However, DNA affects more than just how we look. Some genes contain instructions for controlling when our cells grow, divide, and die.

Exposure to UV radiation can damage DNA. Sometimes this damage affects certain genes that control how and when cells grow and divide. If these genes do not function properly, the affected cells may form a cancer. Most UV radiation comes from sunlight, but some may come from man-made sources such as tanning booths. Scientists have found that the DNA of certain genes is often damaged in melanoma cells. Most of these DNA mutations are not inherited; they are more likely the result of damage caused by UV exposure. Evidence suggests, however, that some people's cells can repair their damaged DNA better than others, and melanoma may be less likely to develop in these people. In the future, better understanding of the way these DNA mutations lead to melanoma may be used to help treat or even prevent this disease.

A mutation in a gene called the *BRAF* gene is found in many melanomas. This mutation is not inherited and seems to occur during the development of the melanoma. Blocking this gene's activity may someday help treat people with advanced melanoma.

In families with inherited, or familial, melanomas, gene mutations that greatly increase the risk of melanoma are passed from one generation to the next. Familial melanomas most often have changes in genes such as *CDKN2A* (also known as *p16*) and *CDK4* that prevent them from controlling the growth of cells as they should. Scientists think that these changes lead to overgrowth and, eventually, to cancer.

Although most moles never turn into melanomas, some do. Researchers have found some changes in DNA that transform benign nevus cells into melanoma cells. It is still not known, however, why some moles become cancerous or why having many moles or atypical moles increases a person's risk of melanoma.

Prevention and Detection

Can Melanoma Be Prevented?

Not all melanomas can be prevented, but there are ways to reduce your risk of melanoma.

Limit Exposure to Ultraviolet Radiation

The most important way to lower your risk of melanoma is to protect yourself from exposure to ultraviolet (UV) radiation. Practice sun safety when you are outdoors. "Slip! Slop! Slap! . . . and Wrap" is a catch phrase that can help you remember the 4 key methods you can use to protect yourself from UV radiation:

- Slip on a shirt.
- Slop on sunscreen.
- Slap on a hat.
- Wrap on sunglasses to protect the eyes and sensitive skin around them.

Protect your skin with clothing

Clothes provide different levels of UV protection, depending on many factors. Long-sleeved shirts, long pants, or long skirts are the most protective. Dark colors generally provide more protection than light colors. Tightly woven fabrics protect better than loosely woven fabrics. Dry fabric is generally more protective than wet fabric.

Be aware that covering up does not block out all UV rays. If you can see light through a fabric, UV rays can get through, too.

Some companies in the United States now make clothing that is lightweight, comfortable, and protects against exposure to UV radiation even when wet. These sun-protective clothes may have a label listing the **ultraviolet protection factor (UPF)** value—the level of protection the garment provides from the sun's UV rays (on a scale from 15 to 50+). The higher the UPF value, the higher the protection from UV radiation.

Newer products, which are used in the washing machine in the same way as detergents, can increase the UPF value of clothes you already own. These products add a layer of UV protection to your clothes without changing the color or texture.

Wear a hat

A hat with at least a 2- to 3-inch brim all around is ideal because it protects areas often exposed to intense sun, such as the ears, eyes, forehead, nose, and scalp. A shade cap also protects these sensitive areas. Often sold in sporting goods and outdoor supply stores, shade caps look like baseball caps with about 7 inches of fabric draping down the sides and back. A baseball cap can protect the front and top of the head but not the back of the neck or the ears, where skin cancers commonly develop. Straw hats are not as protective as ones made of tightly woven fabric.

Use sunscreen

Use sunscreens and lip balms on areas of skin exposed to the sun, especially when the sunlight is strong (for example, high-altitude locations and between the hours of 10 A.M. and 4 P.M.). Many groups, including the American Academy of Dermatology, recommend using products with a **sun protection factor (SPF)** of 30 or more. Use sunscreen even on hazy days or days with light or broken cloud cover because the UV radiation still comes through.

Always follow directions when applying sunscreen. For an average adult, a 1-ounce application (about 2 tablespoons) is recommended to cover the arms, legs, neck, and face. Protection is greatest when sunscreen is applied thickly on all sun-exposed skin. To ensure continued protection, sunscreens should be reapplied every 2 hours. Many sunscreens wash off when you sweat or swim and can be wiped off if you towel dry, so they must be reapplied for maximum effectiveness. Do not forget your lips; lip balm with sunscreen is also available.

According to new labeling rules by the **U.S. Food and Drug Administration (FDA)**, only sunscreens that protect against both UVA and UVB rays may be labeled as "broad spectrum." The new FDA rules also state that only sunscreens that are both broad spectrum and have an SPF of 15 or higher may state that they reduce the risk of skin cancer and early skin aging, when used as directed. These labeling rules are expected to become effective in 2012.

Some people use sunscreen so they can stay out in the sun longer without getting sunburned. Sunscreen should not be used to gain extra time in the sun, because you will still end up with damage to your skin. Sunscreens can reduce your exposure to UV radiation and reduce your risk of melanoma. There is no guarantee, however, and if you stay in the sun a long time, you are at risk for skin cancer even if you have applied sunscreen.

If you want a tan, try using a "sunless" tanning lotion. These products can provide the desired look without the danger. Sunless tanning lotions contain a substance called **dihydroxyacetone (DHA)**. DHA works by interacting with proteins on the surface of the skin to produce color. You do not have to be in the sun for these products to work. The color tends to wear off after a few days.

Wear sunglasses

Wrap-around sunglasses with at least 99% UV absorption provide the best protection for your eyes and the skin around your eyes. Look for sunglasses labeled as blocking UVA and UVB radiation. Labels that say "UV absorption up to 400 nm" or "Meets ANSI UV Requirements" mean the glasses block at least 99% of UV rays. If there is no label, do not assume the sunglasses provide any protection.

Seek shade

Another way to limit exposure to UV radiation is to avoid being outdoors in sunlight too long. Shade is particularly important in the middle of the day between the hours of 10 A.M. and 4 P.M., when UV radiation is strongest. If you are unsure about the sun's intensity, use the shadow test: if your shadow is shorter than you, the sun's rays are at their strongest, and it is important to protect yourself.

When you are outdoors, protect your skin. Keep in mind that sunlight (and UV radiation) can come through light clouds, can reflect off water, sand, concrete, and snow, and can reach below the water's surface.

The UV index: The amount of UV radiation reaching the ground in any given place depends on a number of factors, including the time of day, time of year, elevation, and cloud cover. To help people better understand the intensity of UV radiation in their area on a given day, the National Weather Service and the U.S. Environmental Protection Agency have developed the **UV Index**. This number gives people an idea of the strength of the UV radiation in their area, on a scale from 1 (low) to 11+ (extremely high). A higher number means a higher chance of sunburn, skin damage, and ultimately skin cancers of all kinds. Your local UV Index should be available daily in your local newspaper, on television weather reports, and on the Web site www.epa.gov/sunwise/uvindex.html.

Avoid Tanning Beds and Sunlamps

Many people believe the UV rays of tanning beds are harmless. This is not true. Tanning lamps give out UVA and, usually, UVB rays as well, both of which can cause long-term skin damage and can contribute to skin cancer. Tanning bed use has been linked with an increased risk of melanoma, especially if use is started before the age of 30.

Most dermatologists and health organizations recommend not using tanning beds and sunlamps.

Protect Children from the Sun

Children need special attention because they tend to spend more time outdoors and can burn more easily. Parents and other caregivers should protect children from sun exposure by using the measures already described. Older children need to be cautioned about sun exposure as they become more independent. It is important, particularly in parts of the world where it is sunnier, to cover your children as fully as is reasonable. You should develop the habit of using sunscreen on exposed skin for yourself and your children whenever you go outdoors and may be exposed to large amounts of sunlight.

Children's swimsuits made from sun-protective fabric and designed to cover the child from the neck to the knees are popular in Australia. They are now available in the United States. Babies younger than 6 months should be kept out of direct sunlight and protected from the sun by use of hats and protective clothing.

Sun Exposure and Vitamin D

Doctors are learning that **vitamin D** has many health benefits. It may even help to lower the risk of some cancers. Vitamin D is made naturally by your skin when you are exposed to sunlight. How much vitamin D you get depends on many things, including how old you are, how dark your skin is, and how intensely the sun shines where you live.

At this time, doctors are not sure of the optimal level of vitamin D. A lot of research is being done in this area. It is better to get vitamin D from your diet or vitamin supplements rather than from sun exposure, because dietary sources and vitamin supplements do not increase risk of skin cancer and are typically more reliable ways to get the amount you need.

For more information on how to protect yourself and your family from exposure to UV radiation, contact your American Cancer Society at **800-227-2345** to request the document *Skin Cancer Prevention and Early Detection* or visit our Web site, **cancer.org**.

Identify Abnormal Moles and Have Them Removed

Certain types of moles are at higher risk for developing into melanoma (see the section "What Are the Risk Factors for Melanoma?"). If you have moles, depending on their appearance, your doctor may want to monitor them with regular examinations or may remove them if their features suggest they could be changing into melanoma.

Routine removal of many moles is not generally recommended as a way to prevent melanoma. Some melanomas develop from moles, but most do not. If you have many moles, careful, routine examinations by a dermatologist, along with monthly skin self-examinations, might be recommended.

Any unusual moles or moles that have changed should be checked by a doctor experienced in recognizing skin cancers. See the section "Can Melanoma Be Found Early?" to learn how to recognize suspicious moles and melanoma.

Genetic Counseling and Testing

Gene mutations that increase melanoma risk can be passed down through families, although they account for only a small portion of melanomas. You *might* have an inherited gene mutation that increases your risk of melanoma if any of the following apply:

- several members of one side of your family have had melanoma
- a family member has had more than one melanoma
- a family member has had both melanoma and pancreatic cancer
- you have had more than one melanoma

Genes such as *CDKN2A* (also known as *p16*) are found to be mutated in some families with high rates of melanoma. Tests for these gene changes are now available, although they are not widely recommended by doctors at this time. People interested in learning whether they carry genes linked to melanoma may want to think about taking part in genetic research that will advance progress in this field.

Before getting any type of **genetic testing**, it is important to know ahead of time what the results may or may not tell you about your risk. Genetic testing is not perfect, and the tests may not provide solid answers. Undergoing **genetic counseling** before beginning genetic testing is crucial in deciding whether testing should be done.

Because it is not clear how useful the test results are, most melanoma experts do not currently recommend genetic testing for people with a personal or family history of melanoma. Still, some people may choose to get tested. In any event, people with a family history of melanoma should ask their doctor about getting regular skin examinations, learning to do skin self-examinations, and being careful about sun safety.

Learn More About Skin Cancer Prevention

Many organizations conduct skin cancer prevention activities in schools and recreational areas. Others provide brochures and public service announcements. For more information, see the "Resources" section starting on page 113.

Can Melanoma Be Found Early?

Melanoma can often be found early. Everyone can play an important role in finding skin cancer early, when it is most likely to be curable.

Self-Examination

It is important to check your skin thoroughly, preferably once a month. Learn the pattern of moles, blemishes, freckles, and other marks on your skin so that you will notice any changes. Self-examination is best done in a well-lit room in front of a full-length mirror. A hand-held mirror should be used to help look at areas that are hard to see, such as the backs of the thighs. Examine all areas of your body, including the palms of your hands and soles of your feet, your scalp, ears, nails, and your back. Friends and family members can also help you with these examinations, especially for hard-to-see areas, such as your back.

Be sure to show your doctor any area that concerns you and ask your doctor to examine any areas that are hard for you to see. In men, about 1 of every 3 melanomas occurs on the back. For a more thorough description of a skin self-examination, contact your American Cancer Society at **800-227-2345** and request the documents *Skin Cancer Prevention and Early Detection* and *Why You Should Know About Melanoma*, or visit our Web site, **cancer.org**.

Spots on the skin that are new or changing in size, shape, or color should be evaluated promptly. Any unusual sore, lump, blemish, marking, or change in the way an area of the skin looks or feels may be a **sign** of skin cancer or a warning that it might occur. The skin might become scaly or crusty or begin oozing or bleeding. It may feel itchy, tender, or painful. Redness and swelling may develop. Spots on the skin that look different from the surrounding moles should be evaluated.

It is sometimes hard to tell the difference between melanoma and an ordinary mole, even for doctors, so it is important to show any mole that concerns you to your doctor.

Examination by a Health Care Professional

Part of a routine cancer-related checkup should include a skin examination by a health care professional qualified to diagnose skin cancer. Your doctor should be willing to discuss any concerns you might have about this examination.

Any suspicious lesions or unusual moles should be examined by your primary doctor or by a dermatologist. Many dermatologists use a technique called **dermatoscopy** (also known as dermoscopy, **epiluminescence microscopy [ELM]**, or surface microscopy) to look at spots on the skin more clearly. (See the section "How Is Melanoma Diagnosed?" for more information.)

Normal Moles

A normal mole is usually an evenly colored brown, tan, or black spot on the skin. It can be either flat or raised. It can be round or oval. Moles are generally smaller than 6 mm (about ¼ inch) across (about the width of a pencil eraser). A mole can be present at birth or it can appear during childhood or young adulthood. Several moles can appear at the same time, especially on areas of the skin exposed to the sun. Once a mole has developed, it will usually stay the same size, shape, and color for many years. Moles may eventually fade away.

Most people have moles, and almost all moles are harmless. It is important, however, to recognize changes in a mole that can suggest a melanoma may be developing.

Possible Signs and Symptoms of Melanoma

The most important warning sign for melanoma is a new spot on the skin or a spot that is changing in size, shape, or color. Another important sign is a spot that looks different from all of the other spots on your skin (known as the "ugly duckling sign"). If you have any of these warning signs, have your skin checked by a doctor.

The **ABCD rule** is another guide to the usual signs of melanoma. Be on the lookout and tell your doctor about any spots that match the following description:

- A is for **Asymmetry**: One half of a mole or birthmark does not match the other.
- B is for **Border:** The edges are irregular, ragged, notched, or blurred.
- C is for **Color:** The color is not the same all over and may include shades of brown or black or patches of pink, red, white, or blue.
- D is for **Diameter:** The spot is larger than 6 mm across (about ¼ inch—the size of a pencil eraser), although melanomas can sometimes be even smaller.

Some melanomas do not fit the rules described above, so it is important to tell your doctor about any changes in skin lesions, new skin lesions, or growths that look different from the rest of your moles.

Other warning signs for melanoma include the following:

- a sore that does not heal
- spread of pigment from the border of a spot to surrounding skin
- redness or new swelling beyond the border
- change in sensation—itchiness, tenderness, or pain
- change in the surface of a mole—scaliness, oozing, bleeding, or the appearance of a bump or nodule

Diagnosis and Staging

How Is Melanoma Diagnosed?

If the doctor is concerned that an abnormal area of skin could be skin cancer, certain medical examinations and tests may be used to find out whether it is melanoma, nonmelanoma skin cancer, or some other skin condition. If melanoma is found, other tests may be done to determine whether it has spread to other areas of the body. If you are being seen by your primary doctor and melanoma is suspected, you will likely be referred to a dermatologist, who will examine the area more closely.

Medical History and Physical Examination

Usually, the first step is for your doctor to take your medical history. The doctor will ask your age, when the mark on the skin first appeared, and whether it has changed in size or appearance. You may also be asked about exposures to known causes of skin cancer (including sunburns) and whether anyone in your family has had skin cancer.

During the physical examination, your doctor will note the size, shape, color, and texture of the area(s) in question and whether there is bleeding or scaling. The rest of your body will be checked for spots and moles that could be related to skin cancer.

The doctor may also feel the **lymph nodes** (small, bean-shaped collections of immune system cells) under the skin in the groin, underarm, or neck near the abnormal area. Enlarged lymph nodes might suggest that any melanoma present may have spread.

Along with a standard physical examination, many dermatologists use a technique called dermatoscopy (also known as dermoscopy, epiluminescence microscopy [ELM], or surface microscopy) to examine spots on the skin more clearly. The doctor uses a dermatoscope, which is a special magnifying lens and light source held near the skin. A digital or photographic image of the spot may be taken. When performed by an experienced dermatologist, this test can improve the accuracy of finding skin cancers early. It can help to distinguish benign lesions from cancerous ones without the need for a biopsy.

Skin Biopsy

If the doctor thinks a melanoma might be present, he or she will take a sample of skin from the suspicious area to be examined under a microscope. This procedure is called a skin **biopsy**. Different methods can be used for a skin biopsy. The choice depends on the size of the affected area, where it is on your body, and other factors. Any biopsy is likely to leave at least a small scar. Because different methods produce different types of scars, you should ask your doctor about scarring before the biopsy is done if you are concerned.

Skin biopsies are done with the use of local **anesthesia** (numbing medicine), which is injected into the area with a very small needle. You will probably feel a small prick and a little stinging as the medicine is injected, but you should not feel any pain during the biopsy.

Shave biopsy

A **shave biopsy** is one way to take a skin biopsy. After numbing the area with a local anesthetic, the doctor shaves off the top layers of the skin (the epidermis and the most superficial part of the dermis) with a surgical blade.

A shave biopsy is useful in diagnosing many types of skin diseases and in sampling moles when the risk of melanoma is very low. If melanoma is suspected, however, a shave biopsy is not generally recommended, as the resulting skin sample may not be thick enough to measure how deeply the melanoma has invaded the skin.

Punch biopsy

A **punch biopsy** removes a deeper sample of skin. The doctor uses a tool that looks like a tiny round cookie cutter. Once the skin is numbed with a local anesthetic, the doctor rotates the punch biopsy tool on the surface of the skin until it cuts through all the layers of the skin, including the dermis, epidermis, and the upper parts of the subcutis.

Incisional and excisional biopsies

If the doctor has to examine a tumor that may have grown into the deeper layers of the skin, he or she will use an incisional or excisional biopsy technique. An **incisional biopsy** removes only a portion of the tumor, whereas an **excisional biopsy** removes the entire tumor and is usually the preferred method of biopsy for suspected melanomas.

After numbing the area with a local anesthetic, the doctor uses a surgical knife to cut through the full thickness of skin. A wedge or sliver of skin is removed for examination, and the edges of the wound are sewn together.

Examining the Biopsy Samples

All skin biopsy samples will be looked at under a microscope by a pathologist, a doctor who has been specially trained in the examination and **diagnosis** of tissue samples. Often, the sample is sent to a dermatopathologist, a doctor who has special training in making diagnoses from skin samples.

Biopsies of Melanoma That May Have Spread

Biopsies of areas other than the skin may also be needed. For example, if melanoma has been diagnosed in a skin lesion, the doctor may biopsy nearby lymph nodes to check for metastasis. The types of biopsies discussed in this section may be more involved than those used to sample the skin.

In rare cases, melanoma can spread so quickly that it reaches the lymph nodes, lungs, brain, or other areas before the original skin melanoma is detected. Metastases can sometimes be found long after a skin melanoma has been removed, so it is not clear that it is the same cancer. In some cases, skin lesions go away on their own (without treatment) after cells have spread to other parts of the body. Melanoma can also start in internal organs, although this is rare. In these rare situations, special tests can be done on the biopsy samples to determine whether it is a melanoma or another kind of cancer. For example, melanoma that has spread to the lung could be confused with a primary lung cancer (cancer that starts in the lung). The diagnosis is important because different types of cancer are treated differently.

Fine needle aspiration biopsy

A **fine needle aspiration (FNA) biopsy** is not used on suspicious moles, but it may be used to biopsy large lymph nodes near a melanoma to look for metastasis. This type of biopsy uses a syringe with a thin, hollow needle to remove very small tissue fragments. The needle is smaller than the needle used for a blood test. A local anesthetic is sometimes used to numb the area first. This test rarely causes much discomfort and does not leave a scar.

If the lymph node is near the skin, the doctor can often feel it well enough to guide the needle into it. For a lymph node deeper in the body or an internal organ such as the lung or liver, a computed tomography (CT) scan (a type of x-ray; see page 37) is often used to guide the needle. This test, called a **CT–guided needle biopsy**, can be used if the doctor suspects melanoma has spread to these areas.

FNA biopsies are not as invasive as some other types of biopsies, but in some cases they do not provide a large enough sample to determine whether melanoma is present. In these cases, a more invasive type of biopsy may be needed.

Surgical (excisional) lymph node biopsy

A surgical (or excisional) lymph node biopsy can be used to remove an enlarged lymph node through a small skin incision. Local anesthetic is generally used. This procedure is often done if the size of the lymph node suggests spread of melanoma but an FNA biopsy of the node was not done or did not find melanoma cells.

Sentinel lymph node biopsy

Sentinel lymph node biopsy has become a common way to determine whether melanoma has spread to lymph nodes. The sentinel lymph node is the first lymph node to which cancer will likely spread from the primary tumor. This procedure is used to locate the sentinel node and remove it to check for metastasis.

To map the sentinel lymph node (or nodes), the doctor injects a small amount of radioactive material (and sometimes a blue dye) into the area of the melanoma. After an hour or so, the doctor checks various lymph node areas with a radioactivity detector (which works like a Geiger counter) to see what group of lymph nodes the melanoma is most likely to travel to first. The surgeon makes a small incision in the identified lymph node area. The lymph nodes are then checked to find which one(s) turned blue or became radioactive. When the sentinel node has been found, it is removed and examined under a microscope.

If the sentinel node does not contain melanoma cells, no more lymph node surgery is needed because it is unlikely the melanoma would have spread beyond this point. If melanoma cells are found in the sentinel node, the remaining lymph nodes in this area are removed and looked at as well. This is known as a lymph node dissection.

If a lymph node near a melanoma is abnormally large, the sentinel node procedure may not be needed. The enlarged node is simply biopsied.

Imaging Tests

Imaging tests use x-rays, magnetic fields, or radioactive substances to create pictures of the inside of the body. They are used mainly to look for metastasis to lymph nodes or other organs in the body. They are not needed in people with early-stage melanoma, which is unlikely to have spread.

Chest x-ray

A chest **x-ray** may be done to help determine whether melanoma has spread to the lungs.

Computed tomography

A **computed tomography (CT) scan** is a type of x-ray test that produces detailed, cross-sectional images of your body. Unlike a regular x-ray, CT scans can show the detail in soft tissues, such as internal organs. This test can help determine whether lymph nodes or organs are enlarged, which could be caused by the spread of melanoma. It can also better identify metastasis to the lungs than a standard chest x-ray.

Instead of taking one picture, as does a regular x-ray, a CT scanner takes many pictures as it rotates around you. A computer then combines these pictures into detailed images of the part of your body that is being studied.

Before the scan, you may need to drink a **contrast solution** and/or receive an intravenous (IV) injection of a contrast dye that will help outline abnormal areas in the body. You may need an IV line for the injection of the contrast dye. The injection of contrast dye can cause some flushing (a feeling of warmth, especially in the face). Some people have an allergic reaction to the dye, which can cause hives or, rarely, more serious reactions, such as trouble breathing and low blood pressure. Be sure to tell the doctor if you have ever had a reaction to any contrast material used for x-rays.

CT scans take longer than regular x-rays. You will need to lie still on a table while the scan is done. During the test, the table moves in and out of the scanner, a ring-shaped machine that completely surrounds the table. You might feel a bit confined while the pictures are being taken.

Spiral CT (also known as helical CT) is now available in many medical centers. This type of CT scan uses a faster machine. The scanner part of the machine rotates around the body continuously, allowing doctors to collect the images more quickly than with standard CT. This reduces the chance that images will be blurred because of the patient's breathing motions. Images are more detailed than with a standard CT, and a spiral CT also exposes the person to less radiation.

CT–guided needle biopsy: CT scans can also be used to guide a biopsy needle precisely into a suspected metastasis. For a CT–guided needle biopsy, the person remains on the CT scanning table while a radiologist moves a biopsy needle through the skin and toward the location of the mass. CT scans are repeated until the needle is within the mass. A fine needle biopsy sample (tiny fragment of tissue) or a larger core needle biopsy sample (a thin cylinder of tissue) is then removed to be examined under a microscope.

Magnetic resonance imaging

Like CT scans, **magnetic resonance imaging (MRI)** scans give detailed images of soft tissues in the body. MRIs, however, use radio waves and strong magnets instead of x-rays. The energy from the radio waves is absorbed by the body and then released in a pattern formed by the type of body tissue and by certain diseases. A computer translates the pattern into a detailed image of parts of the body. A contrast material might be injected, as with CT scans, but is used less often. MRI scans are very helpful in looking at the brain and spinal cord.

MRI scans take longer than CT scans—often up to an hour. You may have to lie inside a narrow tube, which is confining and can upset people with a fear of enclosed spaces. Newer, more open MRI machines can help with this if needed. The MRI machine makes loud buzzing noises that you may find disturbing. Some places provide earplugs to help block this noise.

Positron emission tomography

For a **positron emission tomography (PET)** scan, you receive an injection of glucose (a form of sugar) that contains a radioactive atom. The amount of radioactivity used is very low. Cancer cells in the body absorb the radioactive sugar, and a special camera then creates a picture of areas of radioactivity in the body. The picture is not finely detailed like a CT or MRI scan, but it can provide helpful information about your whole body.

This test can be useful to determine whether cancer has spread to the lymph nodes. PET scans are also useful when your doctor thinks the cancer has spread but does not know where. It is most useful in people with advanced melanoma. It is not very helpful in people with early-stage melanoma.

Some newer machines can perform a PET and CT scan at the same time (PET/CT scan), allowing the radiologist to compare areas of higher radioactivity on the PET with the more detailed image of that area from the CT.

Bone scan

A **bone scan** is used to look for cancer that has spread to the bones, but it is rarely used in melanoma. It is only done when other test results or symptoms suggest that the cancer may have spread to the bones.

For this test, a low-level radioactive tracer substance is injected into a vein. Over the course of a couple of hours, the tracer travels through the bloodstream and collects in areas of bone change in the skeleton. You then lie on a table for about 30 minutes while a special camera detects the radioactivity and creates a picture of your skeleton. Areas of bone change, which attract the radioactivity, appear as "hot spots" on your skeleton. These areas may suggest the presence of metastatic cancer, but arthritis or other bone diseases can also cause the same pattern. If an area lights up on the scan, x-rays of the affected area can be done to get a more detailed look. If melanoma is a possibility, a biopsy of the area may be needed to confirm this finding.

How Is Melanoma Staged?

The **stage** of melanoma describes the extent of the cancer in the body. **Staging** is the process of finding out how far the cancer has spread, which includes describing its size as well as whether it has spread to lymph nodes or other organs. The tests described earlier in the section "How Is Melanoma Diagnosed?" are used to help determine the stage of the melanoma.

The American Joint Committee on Cancer (AJCC) TNM system

A staging system is a standard way of summarizing how far a cancer has spread. This system helps members of the **cancer care team** plan appropriate treatment and determine a person's **prognosis,** or outlook.

The system most often used to stage melanoma is the **American Joint Commission on Cancer (AJCC) TNM system**. Several tests and procedures are used to assign T, N, and M categories and a grouped stage. The TNM system for staging contains the following 3 key pieces of information:

- **T** stands for **tumor** (how far it has grown within the skin and other factors). The T category is assigned a number between 0 and 4 according to how far the tumor has grown into the skin. The T category also includes a lowercase letter: "a" if it is not ulcerated or "b" if it is ulcerated. **Ulceration** means the layer of skin covering the melanoma is absent, a detail that can be seen under a microscope after a biopsy.

- **N** stands for spread to nearby lymph **nodes**. The N category is assigned a number between 0 and 3 according to whether melanoma cells have spread to lymph nodes or the lymphatic channels connecting the lymph nodes. It is also assigned a lowercase letter: "a" if melanoma cells can be seen only under a microscope or "b" if they can be seen with the naked eye. The letter "c" is assigned if small areas of melanoma are found in nearby skin or melanoma is found in lymphatic channels around the tumor (but not in the nodes themselves).

- The **M** category is based on whether the melanoma has metastasized to distant organs, which organs it has reached, and sometimes on blood levels of a substance called lactate dehydrogenase (LDH).

There are actually 2 types of staging for melanoma:

- The **clinical stage** is the doctor's best estimate of the extent of disease, based on physical examination, biopsy of the melanoma, and any imaging tests.
- The **pathologic stage** uses all of this information, plus what is found in biopsies of lymph nodes or other organs. Pathologic staging is likely to be more accurate than clinical staging. The clinical stage (which is determined before lymph node biopsy) may actually be lower than the pathologic stage (which is determined after lymph node biopsy).

T categories for melanoma

The T category is based on the thickness of the melanoma and other key factors seen in the skin biopsy. This category is an important part of determining a person's prognosis.

Tumor thickness: The pathologist looking at the skin biopsy measures the thickness of the melanoma under the microscope with a device called a **micrometer**, which is like a small ruler. This technique is called the **Breslow measurement**. Thinner melanomas have a better prognosis. In general, melanomas less than 1 mm in depth (about 1/25 of an inch or the diameter of a period or a comma) have a small chance of spreading. As melanoma becomes thicker, it has a greater chance of spreading.

Mitotic rate: Another important aspect for tumors is the mitotic rate. To measure the **mitotic rate**, the pathologist counts the number of cells that are in the process of dividing (mitosis) in a specified amount of melanoma tissue. A higher mitotic rate (having more cells that are dividing) means that the cancer is more likely to grow and spread. The mitotic rate is used to help stage thin melanomas.

Ulceration: The melanoma tends to have a worse prognosis if there is **ulceration**, meaning the outermost layer of skin is missing.

The possible values for T are as follows:

TX: Primary tumor cannot be assessed.

T0: No evidence of primary tumor.

Tis: Melanoma in situ (the tumor remains in the epidermis).

T1a: The melanoma is less than or equal to 1.0 mm thick, without ulceration, and with a mitotic rate of less than $1/mm^2$.

T1b: The melanoma is less than or equal to 1.0 mm thick. It is ulcerated and/or the mitotic rate is equal to or greater than $1/mm^2$.

T2a: The melanoma is between 1.01 and 2.0 mm thick without ulceration.

T2b: The melanoma is between 1.01 and 2.0 mm thick with ulceration.

T3a: The melanoma is between 2.01 and 4.0 mm thick without ulceration.

T3b: The melanoma is between 2.01 and 4.0 mm thick with ulceration.

T4a: The melanoma is thicker than 4.0 mm without ulceration.

T4b: The melanoma is thicker than 4.0 mm with ulceration.

N categories for melanoma

The possible values for N depend on whether a sentinel lymph node biopsy was done. The clinical staging of the lymph nodes is listed below; it is done without the sentinel node biopsy.

NX: Nearby (regional) lymph nodes cannot be assessed.

N0: No spread to nearby lymph nodes.

N1: Spread to 1 nearby lymph node.

N2: Spread to 2 or 3 nearby lymph nodes OR spread of melanoma to nearby skin or toward a nearby lymph node area (without reaching lymph nodes).

N3: Spread to 4 or more lymph nodes OR spread to lymph nodes that are clumped together OR spread of melanoma to nearby skin or toward a lymph node area and into the lymph node(s).

After lymph node biopsy, the pathologic stage can be determined. The involvement of any lymph nodes can be subdivided as follows:

- Any Na (N1a, N2a, etc.) means that the melanoma in the lymph node is so small that it can be seen only under the microscope.
- Any Nb (N1b, N2b, etc.) means that the melanoma in the lymph node is visible to the naked eye.
- N2c means the melanoma has spread to small areas of nearby skin (satellite tumors) or has spread to lymphatic channels around the tumor (without reaching the lymph nodes).

M categories for melanoma

The M values are as follows:

MX: Presence of distant metastasis cannot be assessed.

M0: No distant metastasis.

M1a: Distant metastases to skin or subcutaneous (below the skin) tissue or distant lymph nodes.

M1b: Metastases to lung.

M1c: Metastases to other organs OR distant spread to any site along with elevated blood LDH level.

Stage Grouping

When a doctor uses the TNM system, he or she will use each letter (T, N, and M) and a corresponding number. For example, a melanoma could be staged as T2a, N0, M0.

To make this information clearer, TNM descriptions are grouped into a simpler set of stages, labeled stage 0 through stage IV. This process is called stage grouping. The stage is described using 0 or Roman numerals from I to IV and is sometimes subdivided using capital letters. In general, people with lower-stage cancers have a better prognosis for a cure or long-term survival.

Stage 0

Tis, N0, M0: The melanoma is in situ, meaning that it involves the epidermis but has not spread to the dermis.

Stage IA

T1a, N0, M0: The melanoma is less than 1.0 mm in thickness. It is not ulcerated and has a mitotic rate of less than $1/mm^2$. It appears to be localized in the skin and was not found in lymph nodes or distant organs.

Stage IB

T1b or T2a, N0, M0: The melanoma is less than 1.0 mm in thickness and is ulcerated or has a mitotic rate of at least $1/mm^2$ OR it is between 1.01 and 2.0 mm and is not ulcerated. It appears to be localized in the skin and was not found in lymph nodes or distant organs.

Stage IIA

T2b or T3a, N0, M0: The melanoma is between 1.01 and 2.0 mm in thickness and is ulcerated OR it is between 2.01 and 4.0 mm and is not ulcerated. It appears to be localized in the skin and was not found in lymph nodes or distant organs.

Stage IIB

T3b or T4a, N0, M0: The melanoma is between 2.01 and 4.0 mm in thickness and is ulcerated OR it is thicker than 4.0 mm and is not ulcerated. It appears to be localized in the skin and was not found in lymph nodes or distant organs.

Stage IIC

T4b, N0, M0: The melanoma is thicker than 4.0 mm and is ulcerated. It appears to be localized in the skin and was not found in lymph nodes or distant organs.

Stage IIIA

T1a to T4a, N1a or N2a, M0: The melanoma is not ulcerated. It has spread to 1 to 3 lymph nodes near the affected skin area, but the nodes are not enlarged and the melanoma is found only when the lymph nodes are viewed under the microscope. There is no distant spread. The thickness of the melanoma is not a factor, although it is usually thick in a person with stage III melanoma.

Stage IIIB

T1b to T4b, N1a or N2a, M0: The melanoma is ulcerated. It has spread to 1 to 3 lymph nodes near the affected skin area, but the nodes are not enlarged and the melanoma is found only when the lymph nodes are viewed under the microscope. There is no distant spread.

T1a to T4a, N1b or N2b, M0: The melanoma is not ulcerated. It has spread to 1 to 3 lymph nodes near the affected skin area. The nodes are enlarged because of the melanoma. There is no distant spread.

T1a/b to T4a/b, N2c, M0: The melanoma may or may not be ulcerated. It has spread to small areas of nearby skin or lymphatic channels around the original tumor, but the nodes do not contain melanoma. There is no distant spread.

Stage IIIC

T1b to T4b, N1b or N2b, M0: The melanoma is ulcerated. It has spread to 1 to 3 lymph nodes near the affected skin area. The nodes are enlarged because of the melanoma. There is no distant spread.

Any T, N3, M0: The melanoma may or may not be ulcerated. It has spread to 4 or more nearby lymph nodes OR to nearby lymph nodes that are clumped together OR to nearby skin or lymphatic channels around the original tumor and to nearby lymph nodes. The nodes are enlarged because of the melanoma. There is no distant spread.

Stage IV

Any T, Any N, M1: The melanoma has spread beyond the original area of skin and nearby lymph nodes to other organs such as the lung, liver, or brain or to distant areas of the skin or lymph nodes. Neither the lymph node status nor thickness is considered in this stage, but typically the melanoma is thick and has also spread to lymph nodes.

Survival Rates for Melanoma By Stage

Survival rates are often used by doctors as a standard way of discussing a person's prognosis. Some people want to know the survival statistics for people in similar situations, whereas others do not find the numbers helpful or do not want to know them.

The **5-year survival rate** and 10-year survival rate refer to the percentage of patients who live *at least* this long after their cancer is diagnosed. Many people live much longer than 5 or 10 years, and many are cured.

In order to get 5- and 10-year survival rates, doctors have to look at people who were treated at least 5 or 10 years ago. Improvements in treatment since then may result in a more favorable prognosis for people receiving a diagnosis of melanoma today.

Survival rates cannot predict what will happen in any particular person's case. Knowing the type and the stage of a person's cancer is important in estimating prognosis. But many other factors can affect a person's prognosis, such as genetic changes in the cancer cells and how well the cancer responds to treatment. Your doctor can tell you if the numbers below apply to you, as he or she is familiar with the aspects of your particular situation.

The following survival rates are based on nearly 60,000 patients who were part of the 2008 AJCC Melanoma Staging Database. These are observed survival rates, meaning they include people with melanoma who died of other causes, such as heart disease. Therefore, the percentage of people surviving the melanoma itself may be higher.

Approximate Survival Rates by Stage

Stage	Approximate 5-year Survival Rate	Approximate 10-year Survival Rate
Stage IA	97%	95%
Stage IB	92%	86%
Stage IIA	81%	67%
Stage IIB	70%	57%
Stage IIC	53%	40%
Stage IIIA	78%	68%
Stage IIIB	59%	43%
Stage IIIC	40%	24%
Stage IV	15% to 20%	10% to 15%*

Survival rate is higher if the spread is only to distant parts of the skin or distant lymph nodes rather than to other organs or if the blood level of lactate dehydrogenase (LDH) is normal.

Other Factors Affecting Survival

Other factors besides stage may also affect survival. For example, older adults generally have shorter survival times. The biggest drop in survival rates begins at age 70. Although melanoma is uncommon among blacks, when it does occur, survival times tend to be shorter than in whites. Some studies have shown that melanoma is more serious if it occurs on a foot, palm, or nail bed. HIV-positive people who have melanoma are also at greater risk of dying of the disease.

Treatment

How Is Melanoma Treated?

Once melanoma has been diagnosed and staged, your cancer care team will recommend treatment options. These options may include one or more of the following:

- surgery
- chemotherapy
- immunotherapy
- radiation therapy

It is important to consider your options carefully. If you do not understand something, ask to have it explained. The treatment options depend largely on the thickness of the primary tumor and the stage of the disease.

Surgery

Surgery is the main treatment option for most cases of melanoma and usually cures early-stage melanoma.

Simple excision

Thin melanomas can usually be cured by a fairly minor surgery called **simple excision**. The tumor is cut out, along with a small amount of normal, healthy skin at the edges, called the **margin**. Local anesthesia is injected into the area to numb it before the excision. The wound is carefully stitched back together afterward. This surgery will leave a scar.

Simple excision differs from an excisional biopsy. The margins are wider in a simple excision because the diagnosis is already known. The margins should be anywhere from 0.5 cm (about ¼ inch) to nearly an inch, depending on the thickness of the tumor. Thicker tumors call for larger margins.

Tumor Thickness and Recommended Surgical Margins

Tumor Thickness	Recommended Margins
In situ	0.5 cm
Less than 1 mm	1 cm
1 to 2 mm	1 to 2 cm
2 to 4 mm	2 cm
Over 4 mm	At least 2 cm

Re-excision (wide excision)

When biopsy confirms a diagnosis of melanoma, the site will often need to be excised again. More skin will be cut away from the melanoma site, and the sample will be viewed under a microscope to make sure that no cancer cells remain in the skin. The size of the margin depends on the thickness of the tumor (see the table above).

If the melanoma is on the face, the margins may be smaller to avoid disfigurement. In some cases, the surgeon may use **Mohs surgery** (although doctors disagree on its use for melanoma). In this procedure, the melanoma and margin is removed layer by layer. Each layer is viewed under a microscope for signs of cancer. The procedure continues until there are no signs of cancer. In theory, this approach allows the surgeon to remove the cancer while saving as much surrounding skin tissue as possible.

Amputation

If the melanoma is on a finger or toe, the treatment may mean **amputation** of all or part of that digit. At one time, some melanomas of the arms and legs were also treated by amputation, but this is no longer done.

Lymph node dissection

In this procedure, the surgeon removes the lymph nodes in the region nearest the primary melanoma. For example, if a melanoma is found on the leg, the surgeon would remove the nodes in the groin region on that side of the body, which is where melanoma cells would most likely travel.

Once melanoma has been diagnosed, the doctor will examine the lymph nodes nearest the melanoma. Depending on the thickness of the melanoma, this may be done by physical examination and/or by imaging tests to look at nodes that are not near the surface.

If the nearby lymph nodes feel abnormally hard or large and a fine needle aspiration biopsy or excisional biopsy finds melanoma in lymph node(s), a lymph node dissection is usually done.

If the lymph nodes are not enlarged, a sentinel lymph node biopsy may be done, particularly if the melanoma is thicker than 1 mm. (See page 36 for a description of this procedure.) If the sentinel lymph node does not contain cancer, it is unlikely melanoma has spread to the lymph nodes and a lymph node dissection is not needed. If the sentinel lymph node contains cancer cells, removing the remaining lymph nodes in that area is usually advised. This procedure is called a complete lymph node dissection.

Before the sentinel lymph node biopsy procedure was developed, surgeons sometimes did a lymph node dissection to determine whether melanoma had spread to nearby lymph nodes. Current treatment guidelines, however, recommend a sentinel lymph node biopsy for this diagnostic purpose.

Although clinical trials are being done in this area, it is not known whether removing lymph nodes that contain melanoma cells improves survival rates. Some doctors feel it could prolong survival and prevent pain that could be caused by cancer growing in the lymph nodes.

A lymph node dissection can cause some long-term **side effects**. One of the most troublesome is called **lymphedema**. Lymph nodes in the groin or under the arms normally help drain fluid from the limbs. If they are removed, fluid may build up and lead to limb swelling, which may or may not go away over time. Elastic stockings or compression sleeves can help some people with this condition. Sometimes special devices that squeeze the limbs are used and may be helpful. For more information about lymphedema, contact your American Cancer Society at **800-227-2345** and request the document *Understanding Lymphedema (For Cancers Other Than Breast Cancer)* or visit our Web site, **cancer.org**.

Because of the risk of lymphedema, as well as the pain from the surgery itself, lymph node dissection is not done unless the doctor thinks it is absolutely necessary. Sentinel lymph node biopsy, however, is unlikely to cause lymphedema. It is important to discuss the possible risks of side effects with your doctor before having these procedures done.

Surgery for Metastatic Melanoma

Once melanoma has spread from the skin to distant organs such as the lungs or brain, the cancer is very unlikely to be cured by surgery. Even when only 1 or 2 metastases are found by imaging tests such as CT or MRI scans, other areas of metastasis are likely to be present that are too small to be found by these scans.

Surgery is sometimes done in these circumstances, although the goal is usually to control the cancer rather than cure it. If one or even a few metastases can be completely removed, surgery may help some people live longer. Removing metastases in some places, such as the brain, might relieve symptoms and improve the person's **quality of life**.

Chemotherapy

Chemotherapy uses drugs that kill cancer cells. Systemic chemotherapy uses drugs that are usually injected into a vein or given by mouth. These drugs travel through the bloodstream to all parts of the body and attack cancer cells that have already spread beyond the skin to lymph nodes and other organs.

Several types of systemic chemotherapy can be used to treat advanced melanoma. Although chemotherapy is usually not as effective in melanoma as in some other types of cancer, it may relieve symptoms or extend survival for some people.

Several of the following chemotherapy drugs may be used to treat melanoma:

- Dacarbazine (also called DTIC) can be used either alone or in combination with other chemotherapy drugs such as carmustine (also known as BCNU) and cisplatin. The combination of these 3 drugs, together with tamoxifen, is called the Dartmouth regimen.
- Another chemotherapy combination used for treating melanoma is cisplatin, vinblastine, and DTIC. This combination is known as the CVD regimen.
- Temozolomide (Temodar) is a drug that works similarly to DTIC, but it can be given in the form of a pill. It may be given by itself, although some studies have shown the drug is more effective when combined with the immunotherapy drug interferon-alpha.
- Paclitaxel is a drug sometimes used to treat melanoma, either alone or combined with drugs such as cisplatin or carboplatin.

It is not clear whether using combinations of chemotherapy drugs is much better than using a single drug. Some studies suggest that combining chemotherapy drugs with 1 or more immunotherapy drugs (interferon-alpha and/or interleukin-2) may be more effective than a single chemotherapy drug alone, although it is not clear if this approach helps people live longer. This type of treatment is also called **biochemotherapy** or **chemoimmunotherapy.**

Isolated limb perfusion: Isolated limb perfusion is a type of chemotherapy sometimes used to treat advanced melanomas that are confined to an arm or leg. It is done during a surgical procedure. Instead of giving chemotherapy intravenously and letting it go throughout the body, this method temporarily separates the blood flow of the involved limb from the rest of the body and injects high doses of chemotherapy into the artery feeding the limb. High doses of chemotherapy can be given to the tumor and surrounding area without exposing internal organs, which would otherwise cause severe side effects. The chemotherapy fluid is usually warmed beforehand, which may help improve its effectiveness. Melphalan is the chemotherapy drug most often used in this procedure.

Possible side effects of chemotherapy

Chemotherapy drugs work by attacking cells that are dividing quickly, which is why they work against cancer cells. Other cells, such as those in the bone marrow, the lining of the mouth and intestine, and the hair follicles, also divide quickly. These cells are also likely to be affected by chemotherapy, which can lead to side effects.

The side effects of chemotherapy depend on the type and dose of drugs given and the length of time they are taken. These side effects may include the following:

- hair loss
- mouth sores
- loss of appetite
- nausea and vomiting
- lowered resistance to infection (because of low white blood cell counts)
- easy bruising or bleeding (because of low blood platelet counts)
- fatigue (because of low red blood cell counts)

These side effects are usually short term and go away once treatment is finished. Some drugs may have specific effects that are not listed above, so be sure to talk with your cancer care team about what you might expect in terms of side effects. There are often ways to lessen side effects. For example, you can be given drugs to help prevent or reduce nausea and vomiting.

Immunotherapy

Immunotherapy stimulates a person's immune system to recognize and destroy cancer cells more effectively. Several types of immunotherapy can be used in treating people with advanced melanoma.

Cytokines for advanced melanoma

Cytokines are proteins that boost the immune system. Two man-made versions of cytokines, interferon-alpha and interleukin-2 (IL-2), are sometimes used in people with melanoma. They are given as intravenous (IV) infusions, at least at first. Some patients or caregivers may be able to learn how to give injections at home. When used alone, both drugs can help shrink advanced (stage III and IV) melanomas in about 10% to 20% of people. These drugs may also be given as part of a biochemotherapy regimen for stage IV melanoma.

Side effects of cytokine therapy may include flu-like symptoms such as fever, chills, aches, severe tiredness, drowsiness, and low blood cell counts. Interleukin-2, particularly in high doses, can cause fluid to build up in the body so that the person experiences swelling and can feel very ill. Because of this and other possible serious side effects, high-dose IL-2 is typically given just in centers that have experience with this type of treatment.

Interferon-alpha as adjuvant therapy

People with melanomas that have penetrated deeply into the skin often have cancer cells travel to other parts of the body. Even if surgery has apparently removed all of the cancer, some of these cells may remain. **Interferon-alpha** can be used as an added therapy after surgery (**adjuvant therapy**) to try to prevent any remaining cells from spreading and growing. Use of adjuvant interferon may delay the **recurrence** of melanoma, but it is not yet clear whether it improves survival.

The interferon must be given in high doses to be effective, but many people cannot tolerate the side effects of high-dose therapy. These side effects can include fever, chills, aches, depression, severe tiredness, and effects on the heart and liver. People taking this drug should be closely monitored by an oncologist who is experienced with this treatment.

People with melanoma and their doctors should take into account the potential benefits and side effects of this treatment when making decisions about adjuvant therapy.

Melanoma vaccines

Vaccines directed at melanoma are being studied in clinical trials. They are experimental, and their benefit is not yet proven. In some ways, these vaccines are similar to the ones used to prevent diseases that are caused by viruses, such as polio, measles, and mumps. Such vaccines usually contain weakened viruses or parts of a virus that cannot cause the disease. The vaccine stimulates the body's immune system to destroy the more harmful type of virus.

In the same way, killed melanoma cells or parts of cells (**antigens**) can be injected as a vaccine in an attempt to stimulate the immune system to destroy melanoma cells in the body. Usually, the cells or antigens are mixed with other substances that help boost the body's immune system as a whole. Unlike vaccines that are meant to prevent infections, however, these vaccines are meant to treat an existing disease.

Making a vaccine that is effective against melanoma has proven to be harder than making a vaccine to fight a virus. Clinical trials are testing the value of treating people with advanced melanoma with vaccines, sometimes combined with cytokine therapy. The results of these studies have been mixed so far, but newer vaccines may hold more promise. For more information on vaccines, see the section "What Is New in Melanoma Research and Treatment?"

Bacille Calmette-Guerin vaccine

Bacille Calmette-Guerin (BCG) vaccine is a bacterium related to the germ that causes tuberculosis. BCG does not cause serious disease in humans, but it does activate the immune system. The BCG vaccine is injected directly into tumors and works more like a cytokine than the melanoma vaccines described earlier, in that it works to enhance the entire immune system. It is sometimes used as part of treatment for stage III melanomas.

Imiquimod cream

Imiquimod (Aldara) is a drug that stimulates a local immune response against skin cancer cells. It is applied as a cream. Some doctors recommend imiquimod for very early (stage 0) melanomas in sensitive areas on the face if surgery might be disfiguring. Not all doctors agree, however, on whether it should be used for melanoma.

The cream is applied anywhere from once a day to 2 times a week for around 3 months. Some people may have serious skin reactions to this drug. Imiquimod is not used for more advanced melanomas.

Radiation Therapy

Radiation therapy uses high-energy rays or particles to kill cancer cells. **External beam radiation therapy** focuses radiation from outside the body on the skin tumor. This type of radiation therapy is used for treating some people with melanoma. The treatment is much like getting an x-ray, but the radiation is more intense. The procedure itself is painless. Each treatment lasts only a few minutes, although the setup time—getting you into place for treatment—usually takes longer.

Radiation therapy is not often used to treat the original melanoma that started on the skin. In some cases, it may be given after surgery in the area where lymph nodes were removed, especially if many of the nodes contained cancer cells. Adjuvant therapy may help reduce the chance that the cancer will recur.

Radiation therapy may also be used to treat melanoma that has recurred in either the skin or lymph nodes or to treat distant spread of the disease. When used to relieve symptoms caused by metastases to the brain or bones, radiation therapy is considered palliative therapy. Palliative radiation therapy is not expected to cure the cancer, but it may help control symptoms.

See the section "What Is New in Melanoma Research and Treatment?" for more information.

Clinical Trials

If you have been told you have melanoma, you have a lot of decisions to make. One of the most important decisions you will make is deciding which treatment is best for you. Maybe someone on your health care team has mentioned a **clinical trial** to you, or you may have heard about clinical trials being done for your type of cancer. Clinical trials are one way to get state-of-the art cancer care. Still, they are not right for everyone.

Here we will give you a brief overview of clinical trials. Talking to your health care team, your family, and your friends can help you make the best treatment choices.

Clinical trials are carefully controlled research studies that are done with patients. These studies test whether a new treatment is safe and how well it works in patients, or they may test new ways to diagnose or prevent a disease. Clinical trials have led to many advances in cancer prevention, diagnosis, and treatment.

Clinical trials are done to get a closer look at promising new treatments or procedures in patients. A clinical trial is undertaken only when there is good reason to believe that the treatment, test, or procedure being studied may be better than the one already being used. Treatments used in clinical trials are often found to have real benefits and may go on to become tomorrow's standard treatment.

Clinical trials can focus on many things:

- new uses of drugs that are already approved by the U.S. Food and Drug Administration (FDA)
- new drugs that have not yet been approved by the FDA
- nondrug treatments (such as radiation therapy)
- medical procedures (such as types of surgery)
- herbs and vitamins
- tools to improve the ways medicines or diagnostic tests are used
- medicines or procedures to relieve symptoms or improve comfort
- combinations of treatments and procedures

Researchers conduct studies of new treatments to try to answer the following questions:

- Is the treatment helpful?
- What is the best way to give it?
- Does it work better than other treatments already available?
- What side effects does the treatment cause?
- Are there more or fewer side effects than the standard treatment used now?
- Do the benefits outweigh the side effects?
- In which patients is the treatment most likely to be helpful?

Clinical trials are usually conducted in distinct phases. Each phase is designed to answer certain questions. Knowing the phase of the clinical trial is important because it can give you some idea about how much is known about the treatment being studied. There are pros and cons to taking part in each phase of a clinical trial.

Phase 0 clinical trials

Even though phase 0 studies are done in humans, this type of study is not much like the other phases of clinical trials. It is included here because some cancer patients may be asked to take part in these kinds of studies in the future.

Phase 0 studies are exploratory studies that often use only a few small doses of a new drug in each patient. They test to find out whether the drug reaches the tumor, how the drug acts in the human body, and how cancer cells respond to the drug. The patients in these studies must have extra biopsies, scans, and blood samples. The biggest difference between phase 0 and the later phases of clinical trials is that there is no chance the patient will be helped by taking part in a phase 0 trial. Because drug doses are low, there is also less risk to the patient in phase 0 studies compared with phase I studies.

Phase 0 studies help researchers find out which drugs do not do what is expected. If there are problems with the way the drug is absorbed or acts in the body, this should become clear very quickly in a phase 0 trial. This process may help avoid the delay and expense of finding out years later in phase II or even phase III clinical trials that the drug doesn't act as expected based on laboratory studies.

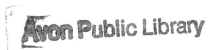

Phase 0 studies are not yet being used widely, and there are some drugs for which they would not be helpful. Phase 0 studies are very small, mostly with fewer than 20 people. They are not a required part of testing a new drug but are part of an effort to speed up and streamline the process.

Phase I clinical trials

The purpose of a phase I study is to find the safest way to give a new treatment to patients. The cancer care team closely watches patients for any harmful side effects.

For phase I studies, the drug has already been tested in laboratory and animal studies, but the side effects in patients are not fully known. Doctors start by giving very low doses of the drug to the first patients and increase the doses for later groups of patients until side effects appear or the desired effect is seen. Doctors are hoping to help the study patients, but the main purpose of a phase I trial is to test the safety of the drug.

Phase I clinical trials are often done in small groups of people with different cancers that have not responded to standard treatment or that recur after treatment. If a drug is found to be reasonably safe in phase I studies, it can be tested in a phase II clinical trial.

Phase II clinical trials

These studies are designed to see whether the drug is effective. Patients are given the most appropriate (safest) dose as determined from phase I studies. They are closely watched for an effect on the cancer. The cancer care team also looks for side effects. Phase II trials are often done in larger groups of patients with a specific cancer type that has not responded to standard treatment. If a drug is found to be effective in phase II studies, it can be tested in a phase III clinical trial.

Phase III clinical trials

Phase III studies involve large numbers of patients—most often those patients who have just received a diagnosis for a specific type of cancer. Phase III clinical trials may enroll thousands of patients. Often, these studies are randomized, which means that patients are randomly put in 1 of 2 (or more) groups. One group (called the **control group**) gets the standard, most accepted treatment. The other group(s) gets the new treatment(s) being studied. All patients in phase III studies are closely watched. The study will be stopped early if many patients experience side effects that are too severe or if one group has much better results than the others. Phase III clinical trials are needed before the FDA will approve a treatment for use by the general public.

Phase IV clinical trials

Once a drug has been approved by the FDA and is available for all patients, it is still studied in other clinical trials (sometimes referred to as phase IV studies). This way, more can be learned about short-term and long-term side effects and safety as the drug is used in larger numbers of patients with many types of diseases. Doctors can also learn more about how well the drug works and whether it might be helpful when used in other ways (such as in combination with other treatments).

What it is like to be in a clinical trial

If you participate in a clinical trial, you will have a team of cancer care experts taking care of you and watching your progress very carefully. Depending on the phase of the clinical trial, you may receive more attention (such as having more doctor visits and laboratory tests) than you would if you were treated outside of a clinical trial. Clinical trials are designed to pay close attention to you. However, there are some risks. No one involved in the study knows in advance whether the treatment will work or exactly what side effects will occur. That outcome is what the study is designed to find out. While most side effects go away in time, some may be long-lasting or even life-threatening. Keep in mind, though, that even standard treatments have side effects.

Deciding to enter a clinical trial

If you would like to take part in a clinical trial, you should begin by asking your doctor if your clinic or hospital conducts clinical trials. There are requirements you must meet to take part in any clinical trial. But whether or not you enroll in a clinical trial is completely up to you. The doctors and nurses conducting the study will explain the study to you in detail. They will go over the possible risks and benefits and give you an **informed consent** form to read and sign. The form says that you understand the clinical trial and want to take part in it. Even after you read and sign the form and the clinical trial begins, you are free to leave the study at any time, for any reason. Taking part in a clinical trial does not keep you from getting any other medical care you may need.

To find out more about clinical trials, talk to your cancer care team. Here are some questions you might ask:

- Is there a clinical trial that I should take part in?
- What is the purpose of the study?
- How might this study be of benefit to me?
- What is likely to happen in my case with, or without, this new treatment?
- What kinds of tests and treatments does the study involve?
- What does this treatment do? Has it been used before?
- Will I know which treatment I receive?
- What are my other choices and their pros and cons?
- How could the study affect my daily life?
- What side effects can I expect from the study? Can the side effects be controlled?
- Will I have to stay in the hospital? If so, how often and for how long?
- Will the study cost me anything? Will any of the treatment be free?
- If I am harmed as a result of the research, what treatment would I be entitled to?

- What type of long-term follow-up care is part of the study?
- Has the treatment been used to treat other types of cancer?

How can I find out more about clinical trials that might be right for me?

The American Cancer Society offers a clinical trials matching service for use by patients, their family, or friends. You can reach this service at **800-303-5691** or on the Web at **http://clinicaltrials .cancer.org**.

Based on the information you give about your cancer type, stage, and previous treatments, this service can put together a list of clinical trials that match your medical needs. The service will also ask where you live and whether you are willing to travel so that it can look for a treatment center that you can get to. You can also get a list of current clinical trials by calling the National Cancer Institute's Cancer Information Service toll-free at **800-4-CANCER (800-422-6237)** or by visiting the NCI clinical trials Web site at **www.cancer .gov/clinicaltrials**.

For even more information on clinical trials, contact your American Cancer Society at **800-227-2345** or visit our Web site, **cancer.org**.

Complementary and Alternative Treatments

When you have cancer, you are likely to hear about ways to treat your cancer or relieve symptoms that are different from standard medical treatment. These treatments can include vitamins, herbs, special diets, acupuncture, or massage—among many others. You may have a lot of questions about these treatments. Talk to your doctor about any treatment you are considering. Here are some questions to ask:

- How do I know if the treatment is safe?
- How do I know if it works?
- Should I try one or more of these treatments?
- Will these treatments cause a problem with my standard medical treatment?
- What is the difference between complementary and alternative treatments?
- Where can I find out more about these treatments?

The terms can be confusing

Not everyone uses these terms the same way, so it can be confusing. The American Cancer Society uses **complementary medicine** to refer to medicines or treatments that are used *along with* your regular medical care. **Alternative medicine** is a treatment used *instead of* standard medical treatment.

Complementary treatments

Complementary treatment methods, for the most part, are not presented as cures for cancer. Most often they are used to help you feel better. Some methods that can be used in a complementary way are meditation to reduce stress, acupuncture to relieve pain, or peppermint tea to relieve nausea. There are many others. Some of these methods are known to help and could add to your comfort and well-being, while others have not been tested. Some have been proven not to be helpful. A few have even been found to be harmful. There are many complementary methods that you can safely use with your medical treatment to help relieve symptoms or side effects, to ease pain, and to help you enjoy life more. For example, some people find methods such as aromatherapy, massage therapy, meditation, or yoga to be useful.

Alternative treatments

Alternative treatments are methods that are used instead of standard medical care. These treatments have not been proven to be safe and effective in clinical trials. Some of these treatments may even be dangerous or have life-threatening side effects. The biggest danger in most cases is that you may lose the chance to benefit from standard treatment. Delays or interruptions in your standard medical treatment may give the cancer more time to grow.

Deciding what to do

It is easy to see why people with cancer may consider alternative treatments. You want to do all you can to fight the cancer. Sometimes mainstream treatments such as chemotherapy can be hard to take, or they may no longer be working. Sometimes people suggest that their treatment can cure your cancer without having serious side effects, and it is normal to want to believe them. But the truth is that most nonstandard treatments have not been tested and proven to be effective for treating cancer.

As you consider your options, here are 3 important steps you can take:

- Talk to your doctor or nurse about any treatment you are thinking about using.
- Check the list of "red flags" below.
- Contact the American Cancer Society at **800-227-2345** to learn more about complementary and alternative treatments in general and to learn more about the specific treatments you are considering.

Red flags

You can use the questions below to spot treatments or methods to avoid. A "yes" answer to any one of these questions should raise a red flag.

- Does the treatment promise a cure?
- Are you told not to use standard medical treatment?
- Is the treatment or drug a "secret" that only certain people can give?
- Does the treatment require you to travel to another country?
- Do the promoters attack the medical or scientific community?

The decision is yours

Decisions about how to treat or manage your cancer are always yours to make. If you are thinking about using a complementary or alternative method, be sure to learn about it and talk with your doctor about it. With reliable information and the support of your health care team, you may be able to safely use methods that can help you while avoiding those that could be harmful.

Treatment of Melanoma by Stage

The type of treatment your doctor recommends will depend on the stage and location of the melanoma and on your overall health. This section lists the options usually considered for each stage of melanoma.

Stage 0

Stage 0 melanomas have not grown deeper than the epidermis. They are usually treated by surgically removing the melanoma and a margin of about ½ cm (about ⅕ inch) of normal skin. For melanomas in sensitive areas on the face, some doctors may use a cream containing the drug imiquimod (Aldara) if surgery might be disfiguring, although not all doctors agree with this use.

Stage I

Stage I melanoma is treated by surgically removing the melanoma, as well as a margin of normal skin. The amount of normal skin removed depends on the thickness of the melanoma. If the melanoma is thinner than 1 mm, a wide excision with a margin of 1 cm (⅖ inch) is recommended. For stage I melanomas with a thickness between 1 and 2 mm, a margin of 1 to 2 cm (⅘ inch) is removed. For stage I melanomas, no more than 2 cm of normal skin needs to be removed from around the tumor. Wider margins make healing more difficult and have not been found to improve survival rates.

Some doctors may recommend a sentinel lymph node biopsy, especially if the melanoma is stage IB or has other characteristics that make metastasis to the lymph nodes more likely. Sentinel lymph node biopsy is an option that you and your doctor should discuss.

Routine lymph node dissection (removal of all lymph nodes near the cancer) is not shown to improve survival in people with stage I melanoma.

Stage II

Wide excision is the standard treatment for stage II melanoma. If the melanoma is between 1 and 2 mm in thickness, a margin of 1 to 2 cm of normal skin will be removed. If the melanoma is thicker than 2 mm, about 2 cm of normal skin is removed from around the tumor site.

Because the melanoma may have spread to lymph nodes nearby, many doctors also recommend a sentinel lymph node biopsy. If a sentinel lymph node biopsy reveals melanoma, the melanoma will be removed and a lymph node dissection (where all the lymph nodes in that area are surgically removed) is done at a later date.

In certain cases (such as if the tumor is found to be thicker than 4 mm or if lymph nodes contain cancer), some doctors may advise use of interferon after surgery. Other drugs or vaccines may also be recommended as part of a clinical trial to try to reduce chances of recurrence.

Stage III

Surgical treatment for stage III melanoma usually requires lymph node dissection, along with wide excision of the primary tumor (as in stage II).

Adjuvant therapy with interferon may help delay recurrence for some people with stage III melanoma.

If several melanomas are present, they should all be removed. If this is not possible, injections of Bacille Calmette-Guerin (BCG) vaccine or interleukin-2 (IL-2) directly into the melanoma is a treatment option. For melanomas on an arm or leg, another possible option is isolated limb perfusion, in which the limb is infused with a heated solution of the chemotherapy drug melphalan. In some situations, radiation therapy is given after surgery in the area where lymph nodes were removed, especially if many of the nodes were cancerous. Other possible treatments include chemotherapy, immunotherapy with cytokines, or biochemotherapy.

Newer treatments being tested in clinical trials may benefit some people. Many people with stage III melanoma will not be cured with current treatments, so they may want to think about taking part in a clinical trial.

Stage IV

Stage IV melanomas are very hard to treat because they have already spread to distant lymph nodes or other areas of the body. Skin tumors or metastases to the lymph nodes that are causing symptoms can often be removed surgically. Metastases in internal organs are sometimes removed, depending on how many are present, where they are located, and how likely they are to cause symptoms. Metastases that cause symptoms but cannot be removed surgically may be treated with radiation, immunotherapy, or chemotherapy.

Current chemotherapy drugs are of limited value for most people with stage IV melanoma. Dacarbazine (DTIC) and temozolomide (Temodar) are the drugs most often used, either alone or combined with other drugs. Even when chemotherapy shrinks these cancers, the effect is often temporary, with an average time of about 3 to 6 months before the cancer starts growing again. In rare cases, however, the chemotherapy is effective for longer periods of time.

Immunotherapy using interferon or IL-2 can help a small number of people with stage IV melanoma live longer. Higher doses of these drugs seem to be more effective, but they also have more severe side effects.

Some doctors recommend biochemotherapy— a combination of chemotherapy and either IL-2, interferon, or both. For example, some doctors are combining interferon with temozolomide. This combination causes more tumor shrinkage, which may make people feel better, although the combination has not been shown to improve survival rates. Another drug combination uses low doses of interferon, interleukin, and temozolomide. Each combination seems to benefit some people. The possible benefits and side effects should be carefully considered before starting any course of treatment.

Because stage IV melanoma is difficult to treat, a person with advanced melanoma may want to think about taking part in a clinical trial. Clinical trials of new chemotherapy drugs, new methods of immunotherapy such as vaccine therapy, and combinations of different types of treatments may benefit some people.

Even though the prognosis for people with stage IV melanoma tends to be poor overall, a small number of people have responded very well to treatment or have survived for many years after diagnosis.

Recurrent Melanoma

Treatment of melanoma that comes back after initial treatment depends on the stage of the original melanoma, the prior treatment, and the site of recurrence. Melanoma may come back in the skin near the site of the original tumor. In general, these local skin recurrences are treated with surgery, similarly to a primary melanoma. Treatment may include a sentinel lymph node biopsy. Other treatments may be considered, depending on the thickness and location of the tumor. These treatments include isolated limb perfusion, systemic chemotherapy, immunotherapy, radiation therapy, or BCG vaccine or interferon.

If nearby lymph nodes were not removed during the initial treatment, the melanoma may come back in these nearby lymph nodes. This symptom may appear as swelling or as a mass. Lymph node recurrence is treated by lymph node dissection and may include adjuvant therapy such as interferon or radiation therapy.

The cancer can also come back in distant sites. Almost any organ can be affected. Most often, the melanoma comes back in the lungs, bones, liver, or brain. Treatment for these recurrences is generally the same as for stage IV melanoma. Melanoma that recurs on an arm or leg may be treated with isolated limb perfusion.

Melanoma that recurs in the brain can be hard to treat. Single sites of recurrence can sometimes be removed by surgery. Most chemotherapy drugs are not able to reach the brain, although temozolomide may be useful. Radiation therapy to the brain may help as well.

As with other stages of melanoma, a person with recurrent melanoma may want to think about taking part in a clinical trial.

Your Medical Team

Your cancer care team comprises several people, each with a different type of expertise to contribute to your care. One of your team members will take the lead in coordinating your care. Most people with skin cancer choose a medical oncologist or dermatologist to lead the team. It should be clear to all team members who is in charge, and that person should inform the others of your progress.

This alphabetical list will acquaint you with the health care professionals you may encounter, depending on which treatment option and follow-up path you choose, and their areas of expertise:

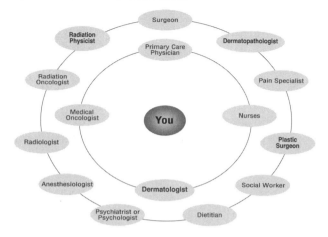

Anesthesiologist

An anesthesiologist is a medical doctor who administers anesthesia (drugs or gases) to render you unconscious or to prevent or relieve pain during and after a surgical procedure.

Dermatopathologist

A dermatopathologist is a doctor specializing in diagnosing skin biopsies under a microscope. He or she will determine the classification (cell type) of your cancer, help determine the stage and grade of your cancer, and issue a pathology report so that you and your doctor can decide on treatment options.

Dermatologist

A dermatologist is a doctor who specializes in the diagnosis and treatment of skin problems.

Dietitian

A dietitian is specially trained to help you make healthy diet choices and maintain a healthy weight before, during, and after treatment. Dietitians can help patients deal with side effects of treatment, such as nausea, vomiting, or sore throat. A registered dietitian (RD) has at least a bachelor's degree and has passed a national competency exam.

Medical oncologist

A medical oncologist (usually called an oncologist) is a doctor you may see after diagnosis. The oncologist is a cancer expert who understands specific types of cancer, their treatments, and their causes. He or she may help cancer patients make decisions about course of treatment and then manage all phases of cancer care. Oncologists most often become involved when you need chemotherapy, but can also prescribe hormonal therapy and other anticancer drugs.

Nurses

During your treatment you will be in contact with different types of nurses.

Case manager: The case manager is usually a nurse or oncology nurse specialist who coordinates the patient's care throughout diagnosis, treatment, and recovery. The case manager provides guidance through the complex health care system by cutting through red tape, getting responses to questions, managing crises, and connecting the patient and family to needed resources.

Clinical nurse specialist: A clinical nurse specialist (CNS) is a nurse who has a master's degree in a specific area, such as oncology, psychiatry, or critical care nursing. The CNS often provides expertise to staff and may provide special services to patients, such as leading support groups and coordinating cancer care.

Nurse practitioner: A nurse practitioner is a registered nurse with a master's degree or doctoral degree who can manage the care of patients with cancer and has additional training in primary care. He or she shares many tasks with your doctors, such as recording your medical history, conducting physical examinations, and doing follow-up care. In most states, a nurse practitioner can prescribe medications with a doctor's supervision.

Oncology-certified nurse: An oncology-certified nurse is a registered nurse who has demonstrated an in-depth knowledge of oncology care. He or she has passed a certification examination. Oncology-certified nurses are found in all areas of cancer practice.

Registered nurse: A registered nurse has an associate's or bachelor's degree in nursing and has passed a state licensing examination. He or she can monitor your condition, provide treatment, educate you about side effects, and help you adjust to cancer, both physically and emotionally.

Pain specialist

Pain specialists are doctors, nurses, and pharmacists who are experts in managing pain. They can help you find pain control methods that are effective and allow you to maintain your quality of life. Not all doctors and nurses are trained in pain care, so you may have to request a pain specialist if your pain relief needs are not being met.

Personal or primary care physician

A personal physician may be a general doctor, internist, or family practice doctor. He or she is often the medical doctor you first saw when you noticed symptoms of illness. This general or family practice doctor may be a member of your medical team, but a specialist is most often a patient's cancer care team leader.

Pharmacist

A pharmacist is a health care professional who dispenses medications and counsels people on their proper use and potential adverse side effects. Pharmacists participate in disease management in collaboration with physicians and other health professionals.

Physician assistant

Physician assistants (PAs) are health care professionals licensed to practice medicine with physician supervision. Physician assistants practice in the areas of primary care medicine (family medicine, internal medicine, pediatrics, and obstetrics and gynecology) as well as in surgery and the surgical subspecialties. Under the supervision of a doctor, they can diagnose and treat medical problems and, in most states, can also prescribe medications.

Plastic/reconstructive surgeon

A plastic surgeon or reconstructive surgeon is a doctor who specializes in reducing scarring or disfigurement that may occur as a result of treatment for diseases, accidents, or birth defects.

Psychologist or psychiatrist

A psychologist is a licensed mental health professional who is often part of the cancer care team. He or she provides counseling on emotional and psychological issues. A psychologist may have specialized training and experience in treating people with cancer.

A psychiatrist is a medical doctor specializing in mental health and behavioral disorders. Psychiatrists provide counseling and can also prescribe medications.

Radiation oncologist

A radiation oncologist is a medical doctor who specializes in treating cancer by using therapeutic radiation. If you choose radiation, the radiation oncologist evaluates you frequently during the course of treatment and at intervals afterward. The radiation oncologist will usually work closely with your oncologist and will help you make decisions about radiation therapy options. A radiation oncologist is assisted by a radiation therapist during treatment and works with a radiation physicist, an expert who is trained in ensuring that you receive the correct dose of radiation treatment. The physicist is also assisted by a dosimetrist, a technician who helps plan and calculate the dosage, number, and length of your radiation treatments.

Radiation physicist

A radiation physicist ensures that the radiation machine delivers the right amount of radiation to the correct site in the body. The physicist works with the radiation oncologist to choose the treatment schedule and dose that will have the best chance of killing the most cancer cells.

Radiologist

A radiologist is a medical doctor specializing in the use of imaging procedures (for example, diagnostic x-rays, ultrasound, magnetic resonance images, and bone scans) that produce pictures of internal body structures. He or she has special training in diagnosing cancer and other diseases and interpreting the results of imaging procedures. Your radiologist issues a radiology report describing the findings to your dermatologist or radiation oncologist. The radiology images and report may be used to aid in diagnosis; to help classify and determine the extent of your illness; to help locate tumors during procedures, surgery, and radiation treatment; or to look for the possible spread or recurrence of the cancer after treatment.

Social worker

A social worker is a health specialist, usually with a master's degree, who is licensed or certified by the state in which he or she works. A social worker is an expert in coordinating and providing social services. He or she is trained to help you and your family deal with a range of emotional and practical challenges, such as finances, child-care, emotional issues, family concerns and relationships, transportation, and problems with the health care system. If your social worker is trained in cancer-related problems, he or she can counsel you about your fears or concerns, help answer questions about diagnosis and treatment, and lead cancer support groups. You may communicate with your social worker during a hospital stay or on an outpatient basis.

Surgeon

Several different types of surgeons provide treatment for skin cancer. A general surgeon is trained to operate on all parts of the body, including the skin. A surgical oncologist is a surgeon who has had advanced training in the surgical treatment of people with cancer. Cancer centers usually have one or more such individuals on their staff.

Although each type of surgeon has a different area of expertise, each plays the same role in treating people with skin cancer. If you require surgery as part of your treatment, the surgeon will perform the operation and then manage any side effects you might have. He or she will also issue a report to your other doctors to help determine the rest of your treatment plan.

More Treatment Information

For more details on treatment options—including some that may not be addressed in this book—the

National Comprehensive Cancer Network (NCCN) and the National Cancer Institute (NCI) are good sources of information.

The NCCN, made up of experts from many of the nation's leading cancer centers, develops cancer treatment guidelines for doctors to use when treating patients. Those guidelines are available on the NCCN Web site (**www.nccn.org**).

The NCI provides treatment guidelines via its telephone information center (**800-4-CANCER**) and its Web site (**www.cancer.gov**). Detailed guidelines intended for use by cancer care professionals are also available on its Web site.

Questions
to Ask

What Should You Ask Your Doctor About Melanoma?

It is important to have honest, open discussions with your cancer care team. They want to answer all of your questions, no matter how minor you might think they are. Consider asking the following questions:

- What type of skin cancer do I have?
- How far has my melanoma spread within or beneath the skin? How thick is my melanoma?
- Are there other tests that need to be done before we can decide on treatment?
- How much experience do you have treating this type of cancer?
- What are my treatment options? What are the possible risks and benefits of each?
- Which treatment do you recommend? Why?
- How long will treatment last? What will it involve? Where will it be done?
- What is my expected prognosis (outlook), based on my cancer as you view it?

- Will I have a scar after treatment? What other side effects might I have?
- What should I do to be ready for treatment?
- What are the chances of my cancer recurring (coming back) with the treatment options we have discussed? What would we do if this happens?
- Should I take special precautions to avoid sun exposure?
- Do I need follow-up appointments to check for recurrence or formation of a new cancer?
- Are my family members at risk for skin cancer? Should I arrange to have my family members screened?

Along with these sample questions, be sure to write down your own questions. For instance, you might want more information about recovery times so you can plan your work schedule. Or you might want to ask about getting a second opinion or about clinical trials for which you may qualify.

After Treatment

What Happens After Treatment for Melanoma?

Completing treatment can be both stressful and exciting. You will be relieved to finish treatment, yet it is hard not to worry about cancer coming back. (When cancer returns, it is called recurrence.) This concern is common among those who have had cancer. It may take some time before your confidence in your own recovery begins to feel real and your fears are somewhat relieved. Even with no recurrences, people who have had cancer learn to live with uncertainty.

Follow-up Care

After your treatment is over, it is very important to keep all follow-up appointments. Follow-up care is needed to check for cancer recurrence or metastasis, as well as possible side effects of certain treatments. This is the time for you to ask your health care team any questions you have and to discuss your concerns.

Your follow-up care should include regular skin and lymph node examinations by you and by your doctor. How often you need follow-up visits depends on the stage of your melanoma at diagnosis. In addition to physical examinations, blood and imaging tests may be recommended for some people.

A typical follow-up schedule for melanomas thinner than 1 mm generally calls for physical examinations every 3 to 12 months for several years. If these examinations are normal, you can return for a checkup once a year. Your doctor may recommend more frequent examinations if you have many moles or a few atypical moles.

For thicker melanomas, a typical schedule might include physical examinations every 3 to 6 months for 2 years, then every 3 to 12 months for the next 2 years. After that, examinations are done at least once a year. Some doctors also recommend chest x-rays (to look for lung metastases) and blood tests (to detect liver or bone metastases) every 6 to 12 months. Other tests such as CT scans may be considered as well, especially for people who had more advanced-stage disease.

It is also important for survivors of melanoma to do regular self-examinations. You should see your doctor if you find a new lump or change in your skin. You should also report any new symptoms that do not go away, such as pain, cough, fatigue, or loss of appetite. Melanoma can come back as many as 10 years after it was first treated. Rarely, melanoma can come back more than 10 years after treatment.

People with stage IV melanoma whose cancer has been removed or has disappeared after treatment usually have the same follow-up schedule as people with thicker melanomas (see page 94). People with persistent stage IV melanoma have a follow-up schedule that is based on their specific situation.

A person who has had one melanoma may still be at risk for another melanoma or nonmelanoma skin cancer. A person cured of one melanoma should continue to examine his or her skin every month and should avoid too much sun exposure.

Seeing a New Doctor

At some point after your cancer diagnosis and treatment, you may find yourself in the office of a new doctor. Your original doctor may have moved or retired, or you may have moved or changed doctors for some reason. It is important that you be able to give your new doctor the exact details of your cancer diagnosis and treatment. Make sure you have the following information:

- a copy of pathology reports from any biopsies or surgeries
- if you had surgery, a copy of your operative report
- if you were hospitalized, a copy of the discharge summary that doctors must prepare when patients are sent home
- if you had radiation therapy, a summary of the type and dose of radiation and when and where it was given
- if you had chemotherapy or immunotherapy, a list of the drugs, dosages, and when they were taken

It is also important to keep medical insurance. Even though no one wants to think of the cancer recurring, it is always a possibility. If it happens, the last thing you want to worry about is paying for treatment.

Lifestyle Changes to Consider During and After Treatment

Having cancer and dealing with treatment can be time-consuming and emotionally draining, but it can also be a time to look at your life in new ways. Maybe you are thinking about how to improve your health over the long term. Some people even begin this process during cancer treatment.

Make Healthier Choices

Think about your life before you learned you had cancer. Were there things you did that might have made you less healthy? Maybe you drank too much alcohol, or ate more than you needed, or smoked, or did not exercise often. Emotionally, maybe you kept your feelings bottled up, or maybe you let stressful situations go on too long.

Now is not the time to feel guilty or to blame yourself. However, you can start making changes *today* that can have positive effects for the rest of your life. Not only will you feel better but you will also be healthier. What better time than *now* to take advantage of the motivation you have as a result of going through a life-changing experience like having cancer?

You can start by working on those things that you feel most concerned about. Get help with those that are harder for you. For instance, if you are thinking about quitting smoking and need help, call the American Cancer Society at **800-227-2345**.

Diet and nutrition

Eating right can be a challenge for anyone, but it can get even tougher during and after cancer treatment. For instance, treatment may change your sense of taste. Nausea can be a problem. You may lose your appetite for a while and lose weight when you do not want to. Some people gain weight even without eating more. This occurrence can be frustrating, too.

If you are losing weight or have taste problems during treatment, do the best you can with eating and remember that these problems usually improve over time. You may want to ask your cancer team for a referral to a registered dietitian, an expert in nutrition who can give you ideas on how to fight some of the side effects of your treatment. You may also find it helps to eat small portions every 2 to 3 hours until you feel better and can go back to a more normal schedule.

One of the best things you can do after treatment is to put healthy eating habits into place. You will be surprised at the long-term benefits of some simple changes, such as increasing the variety of healthy foods you eat. Try to eat at least 5 servings of vegetables and fruit each day. Choose whole-grain foods instead of white flour and sugars. Try to limit meats that are high in fat. Cut back on processed meats like hot dogs, bologna, and bacon. Get rid of them altogether if you can. If you drink alcohol, limit yourself to 1 or 2 drinks a day at the most. And do not forget to get some type of regular exercise. The combination of a good diet and regular exercise will help you maintain a healthy weight and keep you feeling more energetic.

Rest, fatigue, work, and exercise

Fatigue is a very common symptom in people being treated for cancer. Cancer-related fatigue is not an ordinary type of tiredness but a bone-weary exhaustion that does not get better with rest. For some, this fatigue lasts a long time after treatment and can discourage them from physical activity. Exercise can actually help reduce fatigue, however. Studies have shown that people who follow an exercise program tailored to their personal needs feel physically and emotionally improved and can cope better.

If you are ill and need to be on bed rest during treatment, it is normal to expect your fitness, endurance, and muscle strength to decline some. Physical therapy can help you maintain strength and range of motion in your muscles, which can help fight fatigue and the sense of depression that sometimes comes with feeling so tired.

Any program of physical activity should fit your own situation. An older person who has never exercised will not be able to take on the same amount of exercise as a 20-year-old who plays tennis 3 times a week. If you have not exercised in a few years but can still get around, you may want to think about taking short walks.

Talk with your health care team before starting and get their opinion about your exercise plans. Then, try to get an exercise buddy so that you are not doing it alone. Having family or friends involved when starting a new exercise program can give you that extra boost of support to keep you going when the push just is not there.

If you are very tired, though, you will need to balance activity with rest. It is okay to rest when you need to. It is really hard for some people to allow themselves to rest when they are used to working all day or taking care of a household. For more information about fatigue, contact your American Cancer Society at **800-227-2345** and request the document *Fatigue and the Person With Cancer* or visit our Web site, **cancer.org**.

Exercise can improve your physical and emotional health in many ways:

- It improves your cardiovascular fitness.
- It strengthens your muscles.
- It reduces fatigue.
- It lowers anxiety and depression.
- It makes you feel generally happier.
- It helps you feel better about yourself.

Long term, researchers know that exercise plays a role in preventing some cancers. The American Cancer Society, in its guidelines on physical activity for cancer prevention, recommends that adults take part in at least 30 minutes of moderate to vigorous physical activity, above usual activities, on 5 or more days of the week; 45 to 60 minutes of intentional physical activity is preferable. Children and teens are encouraged to try for at least 60 minutes a day of energetic physical activity on at least 5 days a week.

How About Your Emotional Health?

Once your treatment ends, you may find yourself overwhelmed by emotions. This happens to a lot of people. You may have been going through so much during treatment that you could focus only on getting through treatment.

Now you may find yourself thinking about the potential of your own death or about the effect of your cancer on your family, friends, and career. You may also begin to reevaluate your relationship with your spouse or partner. Unexpected issues can also cause concern—for instance, as you become healthier and have fewer doctor visits, you will see your health care team less often. That can be a source of anxiety for some.

This is an ideal time to seek emotional and social support. You need people you can turn to for strength and comfort. Support can come in many forms: family, friends, cancer support groups, church or spiritual groups, online support communities, or individual counselors.

Almost everyone who has been through cancer can benefit from some type of support. What is best for you depends on your situation and personality. Some people feel safe in peer support groups or education groups. Others would rather talk in an informal setting, such as church. Others may feel more at ease talking one-on-one with a trusted friend or counselor. Whatever your source of strength or comfort, make sure you have a place to go with your concerns.

The cancer journey can feel very lonely. It is not necessary or realistic to go it all by yourself. And your friends and family may feel shut out if you do not include them. Let them in   and let in anyone else who you feel may help. If you are not sure who can help, call us at **800-227-2345** and we can put you in touch with an appropriate group or resource.

You cannot change the fact that you have had cancer. What you can change is how you live the rest of your life—making healthy choices and feeling as well as possible, physically and emotionally.

What Happens If Treatment Is No Longer Working?

If cancer continues to grow or returns after one kind of treatment, it is often possible to try another treatment plan that could still cure the cancer or at least help you live longer and feel better. However, when a person has received several different medical treatments and the cancer has not been cured, over time the cancer tends to become resistant to all treatment. When that happens, it is important to weigh the possible limited benefit of a new treatment against the possible downsides, including continued doctor visits and treatment side effects.

Everyone has his or her own way of looking at this situation. Some people may want to focus on remaining comfortable during the time they have left. This is likely to be the most difficult time in your battle with cancer—when you have tried everything medically within reason and it is just not working anymore. Although your doctor may offer you new treatment options, you need to consider that at some point, continuing treatment is not likely to improve your health or change your prognosis.

If you want to continue treatment to fight your cancer as long as you can, you still need to consider the odds of more treatment having any benefit. In many cases, your doctor can estimate the response rate for the treatment you are considering. Some people are tempted to try more chemotherapy or radiation, for example, even when their doctors say that the odds of benefit are less than 1%. In this situation, you need to think about and understand your reasons for choosing this plan.

No matter what you decide to do, it is important that you be as comfortable as possible. Make sure you are asking for and receiving treatment for any symptoms you might have, such as pain. This type of treatment is called **palliative treatment.**

Palliative treatment helps relieve these symptoms but is not expected to cure the disease; its main purpose is to improve your quality of life. Sometimes, the treatments you get to control your symptoms are similar to the treatments used to treat cancer. For example, radiation therapy might be given to help relieve bone pain from bone metastasis. Or chemotherapy might be given to help shrink a tumor and keep it from causing a bowel obstruction. However, this is not the same as receiving treatment to try to cure the cancer.

At some point, you may benefit from **hospice** care. Most of the time, this can be given at home. Your cancer may be causing symptoms or problems that need attention, and hospice focuses on your comfort. You should know that receiving hospice care does not mean you cannot have treatment for the problems caused by your cancer or other health conditions. It just means that the focus of your care is on living life as fully as possible and feeling as well as you can at this difficult stage of your cancer.

Remember also that maintaining hope is important. Your hope for a cure may not be as bright, but there is still hope for good times with family and friends—times that are filled with happiness and meaning. In a way, pausing at this time in your cancer treatment is an opportunity to refocus on the most important things in your life. This is the time to do things you have always wanted to do and to stop doing things you no longer want to do.

Latest Research

What Is New In Melanoma Research and Treatment?

Research into the causes, prevention, and treatment of melanoma is under way in many medical centers throughout the world.

Causes and Prevention

Sunlight and ultraviolet radiation

Recent studies suggest that exposure to ultraviolet (UV) radiation may be linked to melanoma in 2 general ways, although there is likely some overlap.

The first link is to sun exposure as a child and teenager. People with melanoma often have a history of sunburns or other intense sun exposure early in life, although not everyone does. This early sun exposure may start a change in skin cells (melanocytes) that eventually turns them into melanoma cells. Some doctors think this might help explain melanomas that occur on the legs and trunk—areas that generally are not exposed to the sun as much in adulthood.

The second link is to chronic sun exposure, particularly in men. It is thought that this chronic exposure is linked to melanomas that occur on the arms, neck, and face. Tanning booths may encourage either kind of melanoma to develop.

Public education

Most skin cancer can be prevented. The greatest reduction in the number of skin cancer cases and in the pain and loss of life from this disease will come from prevention and early detection strategies. This means educating the public, especially parents, about risk factors for skin cancer. Health care professionals and skin cancer survivors should remind everyone about the dangers of excessive exposure to UV radiation (from the sun and from man-made sources such as tanning beds) and about how easy it can be to protect your skin from too much exposure to UV radiation.

Melanoma should be detected early, when it is most likely to be completely cured. Monthly skin self-examinations and awareness of the warning signs of melanoma may be helpful in detecting most melanomas when they are at an early, curable stage.

The American Academy of Dermatology (AAD) sponsors annual, free skin cancer screenings throughout the country. The American Cancer Society works closely with the AAD to provide volunteers for registration, coordination, and education efforts related to these free screenings. Look for information about screenings in your area or call the AAD for more information. Their telephone number and Web site are listed in the "Resources" section.

The American Cancer Society uses a slogan popularized in Australia as its skin cancer prevention message in the United States. "Slip! Slop! Slap! . . . and Wrap" is a catchy way to remember to slip on a shirt, slop on sunscreen, slap on a hat, and wrap on sunglasses when outdoors to protect your eyes and the sensitive skin around them.

Melanoma DNA research

Scientists have made a great deal of progress during the past few years in understanding how UV radiation damages DNA and how changes in DNA cause normal skin cells to become cancerous. They have also found that DNA damage that affects certain genes is important in causing melanocytes to become cancerous. Sun exposure often causes this damage. Some people, however, may inherit mutated genes from their parents. For example, changes in the *CDKN2A* (*p16*) gene can cause inherited melanoma. People who have a strong family history of melanoma should speak with a genetic counselor or doctor experienced in cancer genetics to discuss the possible benefits, limitations, and disadvantages of testing for changes in this gene.

Molecular staging

Advances in research on DNA and melanoma are also being applied to **molecular staging**. In ordinary staging, a lymph node is removed from the person and examined under a microscope for the presence of melanoma cells. In molecular staging, however, ribonucleic acid, or RNA (a chemical related to DNA), is extracted from cells in the lymph node. Certain types of RNA are made by melanoma cells but not by normal lymph node cells. A sensitive and sophisticated test called **reverse transcription polymerase chain reaction (RT-PCR)** is used to detect these types of RNA.

Early studies have found that RT-PCR is more sensitive than routine microscopic testing in detecting the spread of melanoma to lymph nodes. This test may eventually help identify some people who might benefit from additional treatment, such as immunotherapy, after surgery. However, some doctors are concerned that this test may lead to false-positive results, which might lead doctors to advise unnecessary treatment. That is why this test is not currently recommended. Studies are in progress to learn more about how results should influence choice of treatment.

Treatment

Immunotherapy

Some forms of immunotherapy, such as cytokines (interferon-alpha and interleukin-2) and the BCG vaccine, are already used to treat some melanomas. They work by boosting the immune system in a general way.

Ipilimumab (Yervoy), a newer immunotherapy drug, has been shown to help some people with advanced melanoma live longer. It is just now coming into use, but some doctors may prefer it over other treatment options, such as chemotherapy or other types of immunotherapy.

Ipilimumab targets CTLA-4, a protein that normally suppresses the T-cell immune response, which might help melanoma cells to survive. Researchers are now trying to determine if it might be useful earlier in the course of the disease. Other drugs that counteract CTLA-4 are now being studied as well.

Experimental melanoma vaccines help train a person's immune system to fight melanoma in a more specific way. As researchers learn more about how the immune system works, these immune treatments should become more effective. This is an important area of current research, although melanoma vaccines are currently only available in clinical trials.

In a recent clinical trial of people with advanced melanoma, adding a vaccine to high-dose interleukin-2 (IL-2) increased the portion of tumors that shrank and increased the length of time before tumors started growing again better than IL-2. It is not yet clear whether this vaccine can help people live longer.

Other forms of immunotherapy are also being studied. Some early studies have shown that treating people with high doses of chemotherapy and radiation therapy and then giving them **tumor-infiltrating lymphocytes (TILs)**, immune system cells found in tumors, can shrink melanoma tumors and possibly prolong life. Another study found that T cells (a type of white blood cell) in which genes were altered in the laboratory could cause tumors to shrink in a small fraction of people. Further studies of these new treatments are now under way.

Targeted drugs

As doctors have discovered some of the gene changes in melanoma cells, they have begun to develop drugs that attack these changes. These targeted drugs work differently from standard chemotherapy drugs. They may work in some cases when chemotherapy doesn't. They may also have less severe side effects.

Drugs that target changes in the BRAF gene

About half of all melanomas have changes in a gene called *BRAF*. These changes cause the gene to make an altered *BRAF* protein that signals the melanoma cells to grow and divide. A drug called vemurafenib (PLX4032 or Zelboraf) acts against the altered *BRAF* protein. In studies of people whose metastatic melanoma had a certain *BRAF* gene change (mutation), it caused tumors to shrink in about half of the patients treated. It also seemed to prolong the time before the tumors started growing again and helped patients live longer.

In August 2011, vemurafenib was approved by the FDA to treat advanced melanomas that contain the *BRAF* mutation. This drug is not likely to work in patients whose melanomas have a normal *BRAF* gene, so a sample of your melanoma must be tested to see if it contains the *BRAF* mutation before the drug can be used. This drug is given as a pill, taken twice a day.

The most common side effects seen in the studies of vemurafenib were joint pains, fatigue, hair loss, rash, itching, sensitivity to the sun, and nausea. Serious side effects can occur, such as heart rhythm problems, liver problems, severe allergic reactions, severe skin problems, and severe eye problems. Also, some of the patients treated with vemurafenib in the studies developed new skin cancers, including some melanomas.

Other drugs that target *BRAF* gene changes are now being developed and studied as well.

Drugs that target changes in the c-kit gene

Certain types of melanomas often have unusual gene changes. This often includes melanomas that start in certain areas:

- on the palms of the hands, soles of the feet, or under fingernails
- inside the mouth or in other mucosal areas
- in areas that get chronic sun exposure

About one third of these uncommon melanomas have changes in a gene called *c-kit*. Some drugs that are already used to treat other cancers, such as imatinib (Gleevec) and nilotinib (Tasigna), are known to target cells with changes in *c-kit*. Clinical trials are now under way to see if these and other drugs might help people with these types of melanoma.

Drugs that target other gene or protein changes

Several drugs that target other abnormal genes or proteins, such as sorafenib (Nexavar), bevacizumab (Avastin), temsirolimus (Torisel), and everolimus (Afinitor), are now being studied in clinical trials as well.

Researchers are also looking at combining some of these targeted drugs with other types of treatments, such as chemotherapy or immunotherapy.

Resources

Additional Resources

The American Cancer Society is happy to address any cancer-related topic. If you have questions, please call us at **800-227-2345**, 24 hours a day.

More Information from Your American Cancer Society

The following related information may also be helpful to you. These materials may be ordered from our toll-free number, **800-227-2345**.

Spanish language versions of some of these documents are also available.

A Parent's Guide to Skin Protection

After Diagnosis: A Guide for Patients and Families

Clinical Trials: What You Need to Know

Immunotherapy

Skin Cancer Prevention and Early Detection

Sun Basics: Skin Protection Made Simple (information for children aged 8 to 14)

Understanding Lymphedema (For Cancers Other Than Breast Cancer)

Why You Should Know About Melanoma

National Organizations and Web sites*

In addition to the American Cancer Society, other sources of patient information and support include the following:

American Academy of Dermatology
Toll-free number: 866-503-SKIN (888-503-7546)
Internet: www.aad.org

Environmental Protection Agency
Internet: www.epa.gov/ebtpages/humasunprotection.html

Melanoma Research Foundation
Toll-free number: 800-673-1290
Internet: www.mpip.org

National Cancer Institute
Toll-free number: 800-422-6237 (800-4-CANCER)
Internet: www.cancer.gov

Skin Cancer Foundation
Toll-free number: 800-754-6490 (800-SKIN-490)
Internet: www.skincancer.org

References

American Cancer Society. *Cancer Facts & Figures 2010*. Atlanta, GA: American Cancer Society; 2010.

American Joint Committee on Cancer. Melanoma of the skin. In: Edge SB, Byrd DR, Compton CC. *AJCC Cancer Staging Manual*. 7th ed. New York: Springer; 2010:325–344.

Balch CM, Buzaid AC, Soong SJ, Atkins MB, Cascinelli N, Coit DG, Fleming ID, Gershenwald JE, Houghton A Jr, Kirkwood JM, McMasters KM, Mihm MF, Morton DL, Reintgen DS, Ross MI, Sober A, Thompson JA, Thompson JF. Final version of the American Joint Committee on Cancer

*Inclusion on this list does not imply endorsement by the American Cancer Society.

staging system for cutaneous melanoma. *J Clin Oncol.* 2001;19(16):3635–3648. (See also pages 3622–3634.)

Berman B, Villa AM. Immune response modulators in the treatment of skin cancer. In: Rigel DS, Friedman RJ, Dzubow LM, Reintgen DS, Bystryn JC, Marks R, eds. *Cancer of the Skin.* Philadelphia, PA: Elsevier Saunders; 2005:499–513.

Cormier JN, Xing Y, Ding M, Lee JE, Mansfield PF, Gershenwald JE, Ross MI, Du XL. Population-based assessment of surgical treatment trends for patients with melanoma in the era of sentinel lymph node biopsy. *J Clin Oncol.* 2005;23(25):6054–6052.

Curtin JA, Fridlyand J, Kageshita T, Patel HN, Busam KJ, Kutzner H, Cho KH, Aiba S, Bröcker EB, LeBoit PE, Pinkel D, Bastian BC. Distinct sets of genetic alterations in melanoma. *N Engl J Med.* 2005;353(20):2135–2147.

Dudley ME, Yang JC, Sherry R, Hughes MS, Royal R, Kammula U, Robbins PF, Huang J, Citrin DE, Leitman SF, Wunderlich J, Restifo NP, Thomasian A, Downey SG, Smith FO, Klapper J, Morton K, Laurencot C, White DE, Rosenberg SA. Adoptive cell therapy for patients with metastatic melanoma: evaluation of intensive myeloablative chemoradiation preparative regimens. *J Clin Oncol.* 2008;26(32):5233–5239.

El Ghissassi F, Baan R, Straif K, Grosse Y, Secretan B, Bouvard V, Benbrahim-Tallaa L, Guha N, Freeman C, Galichet L, Cogliano V; WHO International Agency for Research on Cancer Monograph Working Group. A review of human carcinogens—part D: radiation. *Lancet Oncol.* 2009;10(8):751–752.

Horner MJ, Ries LAG, Krapcho M, Neyman N, Aminou R, Howlader N, Altekruse SF, Feuer EJ, Huang L, Mariotto A, Miller BA, Lewis DR, Eisner MP,

Stinchcomb DG, Edwards BK (eds). *SEER Cancer Statistics Review, 1975–2006*, National Cancer Institute. Bethesda, MD, http://seer.cancer.gov/csr/1975_2006/, based on November 2008 SEER data submission, posted to the SEER web site, 2009.

Huang CL, Halpern AC. Management of the patient with melanoma. In: Rigel DS, Friedman RJ, Dzubow LM, Reintgen DS, Bystryn JC, Marks R, eds. *Cancer of the Skin*. Philadelphia, PA: Elsevier Saunders; 2005:265–273.

Lange JR, Fecher LA, Sharfman WH, et al. Melanoma. In: Abeloff MD, Armitage JO, Niederhuber JE. Kastan MB, McKenna WG, eds. *Abeloff's Clinical Oncology*. 4th ed. Philadelphia, PA: Elsevier; 2008:1229–1252.

Leachman SA, Lowstuter K, Wadge LM. Genetic testing for melanoma. In: Rigel DS, Friedman RJ, Dzubow LM, Reintgen DS, Bystryn JC, Marks R, eds. *Cancer of the Skin*. Philadelphia, PA: Elsevier Saunders; 2005:281–290.

Morgan RA, Dudley ME, Wunderlich JR, Hughes MS, Yang JC, Sherry RM, Royal RE, Topalian SL, Kammula US, Restifo NP, Zheng Z, Nahvi A, de Vries CR, Rogers-Freezer LJ, Mavroukakis SA, Rosenberg SA. Cancer regression in patients after transfer of genetically engineered lymphocytes. *Science*. 2006;314(5796):126–129.

National Cancer Institute. Physician Data Query (PDQ). *Melanoma Treatment. 2009*. National Cancer Institute Web site. www.cancer.gov/cancertopics/pdq/treatment/melanoma/HealthProfessional. Accessed August 10, 2009.

National Comprehensive Cancer Network (NCCN). *Practice Guidelines in Oncology: Melanoma*. Version 2.2009. National Comprehensive Cancer Network Web site. www.nccn.org/professionals/

physician_gls/PDF/melanoma.pdf. Accessed August 10, 2009.

Schwartzentruber DJ, Lawson D, Richards J, Condry RM, Miller D, Triesman J, Gailani F, Riley B, Vena D, Hwu P. A phase III multi-institutional randomized study of immunization with the gp100.209–217(210M) peptide followed by high-dose IL-2 compared with high-dose IL-2 alone in patients with metastatic melanoma. *J Clin Oncol.* 2009;27:18s (suppl; abstr CRA9011).

Slingluff CL, Flaherty K, Rosenberg SA, Read PW. Cutaneous melanoma. In: DeVita VT, Lawrence TS, Rosenberg SA, eds. *DeVita, Hellman, and Rosenberg's Cancer: Principles and Practice of Oncology.* 8th ed. Philadelphia, PA: Lippincott Williams & Wilkins; 2008:1897–1951.

Thompson JF, Scolyer RA, Kefford RF. Cutaneous melanoma. *Lancet.* 2005;365(9460):687–701.

Tsao H, Atkins MB, Sober AJ. Management of cutaneous melanoma. *N Engl J Med.* 2004;351(10):998–1012. Erratum in: *N Engl J Med.* 2004 Dec 2; 351(23):2461.

Glossary

ABCD rule: a list of traits that should be considered when distinguishing a normal mole from one that should be checked by a doctor:

> **Asymmetry:** One half of the mole does not match the other half.
>
> **Border irregularity:** The edges of the mole are irregular, ragged, blurred, or notched.
>
> **Color:** The color of the mole is not the same all over. There may be different shades of tan, brown, or black and sometimes patches of pink, red, blue, or white.
>
> **Diameter:** The mole is larger than 6 mm across (about ¼ inch or about the size of a pencil eraser) although melanomas can sometimes be smaller than this.

adjuvant (AJ-uh-vunt) therapy: additional treatment given after the main treatment. It usually refers to hormone therapy, chemotherapy, radiation therapy, or immunotherapy added after surgery to increase the chances of curing the disease or prevent it from coming back.

AJCC staging system: *see* American Joint Committee on Cancer staging system.

alternative medicine (alternative therapy): an unproven medication or therapy that is recommended instead of standard (proven) therapy. Some alternative therapies have dangerous or even life-threatening side effects. With others, the main danger is that the patient may lose the opportunity to benefit from standard therapy. The American Cancer Society recommends that patients considering the use of any alternative or complementary therapies discuss them with their cancer care team. *Compare with* complementary medicine.

American Joint Committee on Cancer (AJCC) TNM staging system: a system for describing the extent of a cancer's spread by using 0 and the Roman numerals I through IV. Also called the TNM system. *See also* staging.

amputation: surgery to remove part or all of a limb or appendage.

anesthesia: the loss of feeling or sensation as a result of drugs or gases. **General anesthesia** causes loss of consciousness (puts you to sleep). **Local** or **regional anesthesia** numbs only a certain area of the body. *See also* anesthetic.

anesthetic: a topical or intravenous substance that causes loss of feeling or awareness in a part of the body. General anesthetics are used to put patients to sleep for procedures. *See also* anesthesia.

antibody: a protein produced by the body's immune system cells and released into the blood. Antibodies defend the body against foreign agents, such as bacteria. These agents contain certain substances called antigens. Each antibody works against a specific antigen. *See also* antigen.

antigen: a substance that causes the body's immune system to react. This reaction often involves production of antibodies. For example, the immune system's response to antigens that are part of bacteria and viruses helps people resist infections. Cancer cells have certain antigens that can be found by laboratory tests. Other cancer cell antigen's play a role in immune reactions that may help the body's resistance to cancer. *See also* antibody.

Bacille Calmette-Guerin vaccine (BCG): an effective immunization against tuberculosis. Commonly abbreviated BCG, it is an weakened version of a bacterium called Mycobacterium bovis, which is closely related to Mycobacterium tuberculosis, the agent responsible for tuberculosis. This vaccine is also used in the treatment for some types of skin cancers.

basal cell: a small, round cell found in the lower part (or base) of the epidermis, the outer layer of the skin.

basal cell cancer: *see* basal cell carcinoma.

basal cell carcinoma: a type of skin cancer that arises from the basal cells, small round cells found in the lower part (or base) of the epidermis, the outer layer of the skin.

basement membrane: a very thin layer of tissue upon which is posed a single layer of cells. The basement membrane is made up of proteins held together by collagen. *See also* collagen.

benign: not cancer; not malignant.

biochemotherapy: the use of immunotherapy in conjunction with chemotherapy. Also called chemoimmunotherapy. *See* chemotherapy, immunotherapy.

biopsy: the removal of a sample of tissue to see whether cancer cells are present. There are several kinds of biopsies. *See also* fine needle aspiration biopsy and CT–guided needle biopsy.

> **excisional biopsy:** a surgical procedure in which an entire lump or suspicious area is removed for diagnosis. The tissue is then examined under a microscope.
> **incisional biopsy:** a surgical procedure in which a portion of a lump or suspicious area is removed for diagnosis. The tissue is then examined under a microscope.
> **punch biopsy:** removal of a small disk-shaped sample of tissue by use of a sharp, hollow device. The tissue is then examined under a microscope.
> **shave biopsy:** a procedure in which a skin abnormality and a thin layer of surrounding skin are removed with a small blade for examination under a microscope.

bone scan: an imaging method that gives important information about the bones, including the location of cancer that may have spread to the bones. It can be done as an outpatient procedure and is painless, except for the needle stick when a low-dose radioactive substance is injected into a vein. Special pictures are taken to see where the radioactivity collects, pointing to an abnormality. *See also* imaging tests.

Breslow measurement: a measurement showing the actual thickness of the tumor under a microscope by of a tiny measuring device.

cancer: cancer is not just one disease but a group of diseases. All forms of cancer cause cells in the body to change and grow out of control. Most types of cancer cells form a lump or mass called a tumor. The tumor can invade and destroy healthy tissue. Cells from the tumor can break away and travel to other parts of the body, where they can continue to grow. This spreading process is called metastasis. When cancer spreads, it is still named after the part of the body where it started. For example, if breast cancer spreads to the lungs, it is still called breast cancer, not lung cancer.

Some cancers, such as blood cancers, do not form a tumor. Not all tumors are cancer. A tumor that is not cancer is called benign. Benign tumors do not grow and spread the way cancer does. Benign tumors are usually not a threat to life. Another word for cancerous is malignant.

cancer care team: the group of health care professionals who work together to identify, treat, and care for people with cancer. The cancer care team may include the following and others: primary care physicians, pathologists, oncology specialists (medical oncologist, radiation oncologist), surgeons, nurses, oncology nurse specialists, and oncology social workers. Whether the team is linked formally or informally, there is usually one person who takes the job of coordinating the team.

cancer cell: a cell that divides and reproduces abnormally and has the potential to spread throughout the body, crowding out normal cells and tissue. *See also* metastasis, cancer.

cell: the basic unit of which all living things are made. Cells replace themselves by splitting and forming new cells (mitosis). The processes that control the formation of new cells and the death of old cells are disrupted in cancer.

chemoimmunotherapy: chemotherapy combined with immunotherapy. Chemotherapy uses different drugs to kill or slow the growth of cancer cells; immunotherapy uses treatments to stimulate or restore the ability of the immune system to fight cancer. Also called biochemotherapy.

chemotherapy: treatment with drugs to destroy cancer cells. Chemotherapy is often used, either alone or with surgery or radiation, to treat cancer that has spread or recurred, or when there is a strong chance that it could recur. *See also* systemic therapy.

clinical stage: an estimate of the extent of cancer based on physical examination, biopsy results, and imaging tests. *See also* pathologic stage, molecular staging, staging.

clinical trials: research studies to test new drugs or treatments to compare current, standard treatments with others that may be better. Before a new treatment is used on people, it is studied in the laboratory. If laboratory studies suggest the treatment will work, the next step is to test its value for patients. These human studies are called clinical trials. *See also* control group.

collagen: a fibrous protein that is the major constituent of cartilage and other connective tissue.

complementary medicine (complementary therapy): treatment used in addition to standard therapy. Some complementary therapies may help relieve certain symptoms of cancer, relieve side effects of standard cancer therapy, or improve a person's sense of well-being. The American Cancer Society recommends that patients considering the use of any alternative or complementary therapies discuss these therapies with their cancer care team, since many of these treatments are unproven and some can be harmful. *Compare with* alternative medicine.

computed tomography (to-MAHG-ruh-fee) scan: an imaging test in which many x-rays are taken of a part of the body from different angles. These images are combined by a computer to produce cross-sectional pictures of internal organs. Except for the injection of a contrast dye (needed in some but not all cases), this is a painless procedure that can be done in an outpatient clinic. It is often referred to as a "CT" or "CAT" scan.

congenital melanocytic nevi: benign growths (usually brown or black) on the skin that are formed by a cluster of melanocytes. Congenital melanocytic nevi are present at birth or develop in the first year or so of life. *See also* nevus, mole, melanocyte.

contrast solution: any material used in imaging tests, such as x-rays and MRI and CT scans, to help outline the body parts being examined. These solutions may be injected or ingested (drunk). Also called contrast dye, radiocontrast dye, radiocontrast medium.

control group: in research or clinical trials, the group that does not receive the treatment being tested. The group may get a placebo or sham treatment, or it may receive standard therapy. Also called the comparison group. *See also* clinical trials.

CT–guided needle biopsy: a procedure that uses special x-rays to locate a mass, while the radiologist advances a biopsy needle toward it. The images are repeated until the doctor is sure the needle is in the tumor or mass. A small sample of tissue is then taken from the mass to be examined under a microscope. *See also* biopsy.

CT scan or CAT scan: *see* computed tomography.

cytokine (SY-toh-kine): a product of cells of the immune system that may stimulate immunity and cause regression of some cancers. Cytokines can also be produced in the laboratory and given to people to affect immune responses.

dermatoscopy: an examination technique that uses a hand-held skin surface microscope. The skin surface is illuminated by a halogen bulb and the glass disc of the scope is pressed against the skin, making details of the epidermis become visible. Also known as dermoscopy. *See also* epiluminescence microscopy (ELM).

dermis: the lower or inner layer of the two main layers of tissue that make up the skin.

diagnosis: identifying a disease by its signs or symptoms and by using imaging procedures and laboratory findings. For some types of cancer, the earlier a diagnosis is made, the better the chance for long-term survival.

dihydroxyacetone (DHA): the active chemical ingredient in sunless tanning lotions. When applied to the skin, DHA reacts with the amino acids in the skin and causes the pigment to darken.

DNA: deoxyribonucleic acid. DNA is the genetic "blueprint" found in the nucleus of each cell. It holds genetic information on cell growth, division, and function.

dysplastic nevus: a type of nevus (mole) that looks different from a common mole. A dysplastic nevus is often larger with borders that are not easy to see. Its color is usually uneven and can range from pink to dark brown. Parts of the mole may be raised above the skin surface. A dysplastic nevus may develop into malignant melanoma.

epidermis: the upper or outer layer of the two main layers of tissue that make up the skin.

epiluminescence microscopy (ELM): a technique that uses a hand-held magnifying lens to examine the skin and determine whether cancer is present in pigmented skin lesions. *See also* dermatoscopy.

excisional biopsy: *see* biopsy.

external beam radiation therapy (EBRT): radiation that is focused from a source outside the body on the area affected by the cancer. It is much like getting a diagnostic x-ray, but for a longer period.

FDA: *see* U.S. Food and Drug Administration.

fibroblast: a connective tissue cell that makes and secretes collagen proteins. *See also* collagen.

fine needle aspiration biopsy: a procedure in which a thin needle is used to draw up (aspirate) samples for examination under a microscope. *See also* biopsy.

first-degree relative: a parent, sibling, or child.

five (5)-year survival rate: the percentage of people with a given cancer who are expected to survive 5 years or longer with the disease. Five-year survival rates have some drawbacks. Although the rates are based on the most recent information available, they may include data from patients treated several years earlier. Advances in cancer treatment often occur quickly. Five-year survival rates, while statistically valid, may not reflect these advances. They should not be seen as a predictor in an individual case.

gene: a segment of DNA that contains information on hereditary characteristics such as hair color, eye color, and height, as well as susceptibility to certain diseases. *See also* DNA, genetic risk factor, genetic counseling, genetic testing.

gene therapy: treatment that alters a gene. In studies of gene therapy for cancer, researchers are trying to improve the body's natural ability to fight the disease or to make the cancer cells more sensitive to other kinds of therapy.

genetic counseling: the process of counseling people who may have a gene that makes them more susceptible to cancer. The purpose of the counseling is to help them decide whether they wish to be tested, to explore what the genetic test results might mean, and to support them before and after the test. *See also* gene, genetic testing, genetic risk factor.

genetic risk factor: a risk factor that is inherited from a parent. A risk factor is anything that increases a person's chance of getting a disease such as cancer. Risk factors can be lifestyle-related or environmental, or genetic (inherited). Having a risk factor, or several risk factors, does not mean that a person will get the disease. Most cancers are not caused by genetic risk factors. If a patient has several family members with cancer, however, genetic testing may be considered. *See also* gene, risk factor, genetic testing, genetic counseling.

genetic testing: tests performed to see if a person has certain gene changes known to increase cancer risk. Such testing is not recommended for everyone, rather for those with specific types of family history. Genetic counseling should be part of the process. *See also* gene, genetic counselor, genetic risk factor.

hemangioma: abnormal buildup of blood vessels in the skin or internal organs.

hospice: a special kind of care for people in the final phase of illness, their families, and caregivers. The care may take place in the person's home or in a home-like facility. The focus is on comfort, not cure.

imaging tests: methods used to produce pictures of internal body structures. Some imaging methods used to help diagnose or stage cancer are x-rays, CT scans, magnetic resonance imaging (MRI), and ultrasound.

immunotherapy: treatment to boost or restore the ability of the immune system to fight cancer, infections, and other diseases. Also used to lessen certain side effects that may be caused by some cancer treatments. Agents used in immunotherapy include monoclonal antibodies, growth factors, and vaccines. These agents may also have a direct antitumor effect. Also called biological response modifier therapy, biological therapy, biotherapy, and BRM therapy.

incisional biopsy: *see* biopsy.

informed consent: a legal document that explains a course of treatment, the risks, benefits, and possible alternatives; the process by which patients agree to treatment.

interferon-alpha: a type of immunotherapy that uses a synthetic protein that resembles a protein that occurs naturally in the body. Interferon is given as an injection just under the skin, usually in the thigh or abdomen. Interferon is given to slow down or stop cancer cells dividing, to reduce the ability of cancer cells to protect themselves from the immune system, and to strengthen the body's immune system. *See also* immunotherapy.

isolated limb perfusion: a procedure that may be used to deliver anticancer drugs directly to an arm or leg. The flow of blood to and from the limb is temporarily stopped with a tourniquet (a tight band around the limb), and anticancer drugs are put directly into the blood of the limb. This procedure allows the person to receive a high dose of drugs in the area where the cancer occurred. Also called limb perfusion.

keratin: a tough, insoluble protein found in the outer layer of the skin.

keratinocytes: cells found in the outer layer of the skin that produce keratin, a tough insoluble protein.

lipoma: a benign tumor made of fat cells.

lymphedema: swelling due to a collection of excess fluid in the arms or legs. This may happen after the lymph nodes and vessels are removed or are injured by radiation, or it can happen many years after treatment. It may also happen when a tumor disrupts normal fluid drainage. Lymphedema can persist and interfere with activities of daily living. *See also* lymph nodes.

lymph nodes: small, bean-shaped collections of immune system tissue that are found along lymphatic vessels. They remove cell waste, germs, and other harmful substances from lymph. They help fight infections and also have a role in fighting cancer, although cancers sometimes spread through lymph nodes. Also called lymph glands.

lymphocyte: a type of white blood cell that helps the body fight infection.

magnetic resonance imaging (MRI): a method of taking pictures of the inside of the body. Instead of using x-rays,

MRI uses a powerful magnet to send radio waves through the body. The images appear on a computer screen, as well as on film. Like x-rays, the procedure is physically painless, but some people may feel confined inside the MRI machine, and it is noisy.

malignant: cancerous.

margin: the edge of the cancerous tissue removed during surgery. A negative surgical margin is a sign that no cancer was left behind. A positive surgical margin means that cancer cells are found at the outer edge of the removed sample, and is usually a sign that some cancer is still in the body.

melanin: a pigment that gives color to skin and eyes and helps protect them from damage by ultraviolet rays.

melanocyte: a type of cell in the skin and eyes that produces and contains the pigment called melanin.

melanoma: a form of cancer that begins in melanocytes. It may begin in a mole (skin melanoma), but can also begin in other pigmented tissues, such as in the eye or in the intestines.

Merkel cell carcinoma: a rare type of skin cancer that usually appears as a flesh-colored or bluish-red nodule, often on the face, head, or neck. Merkel cell carcinoma tends to grow fast and spread quickly to other parts of the body. It is named after the Merkel cell, which is found at the base of the epidermis, the outermost layer of the skin. *See also* Merkel cell polyomavirus.

Merkel cell polyomavirus (MCV): the virus that is suspected to cause most cases of Merkel cell carcinoma.

metastasis: the spread of cancer cells from one part of the body to another, often by way of the lymphatic system or bloodstream. **Regional metastasis** is the spread of cancer to the lymph nodes, tissues, or organs close to the primary site. **Distant metastasis** is the spread of cancer to organs or tissues that are farther away (such as

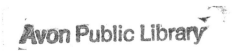

when skin cancer spreads to the lungs). The plural of this word is metastases. *See also* lymph nodes, metastasize, metastatic.

metastasize (meh-TAS-tuh-size): the spread of cancer cells to one or more sites elsewhere in the body, often by way of the lymphatic system or bloodstream. *See also* metastasis.

metastatic (met-uh-STAT-ick) cancer: pertaining to the spread of cancer from the primary site (where it started) to other structures or organs, nearby or far away. *See also* metastasis, metastasize.

micrometer: a unit of measure equal to one-millionth of a meter.

mitotic rate: the speed at which the cells divide. Cancer tissue generally has a higher mitotic rate than normal tissues.

Mohs surgery: a surgical procedure used to treat skin cancer. Individual layers of cancerous tissue are removed and examined under a microscope one at a time until all cancerous tissue has been removed. Also called Mohs micrographic surgery.

mole: a benign (noncancerous) growth on the skin that is formed by a cluster of melanocytes (cells that make a substance called melanin, which gives color to skin and eyes). A mole is usually dark and may be raised from the skin. Also called nevus.

molecular staging: the process of staging a disease by studying molecules, such as proteins, DNA, and RNA, in a tissue or fluid. *See also* pathologic stage, clinical stage, staging.

MRI: *see* magnetic resonance imaging.

mutations: permanent changes in the DNA of a cell caused by exposure to damaging agents in the environment or mistakes made during cell division (mitosis). Mutations may be harmful, beneficial, or have no effect. Certain mutations may lead to cancer or other disease. *See also* DNA.

nevus (NEE-vus): a benign (noncancerous) growth on the skin that is formed by a cluster of melanocytes (cells that make a substance called melanin, which gives color to skin and eyes). A nevus is usually dark and may be raised from the skin. Also called mole. *See also* melanocyte, melanin.

nonmelanoma skin cancer: skin cancer that forms in basal cells or squamous cells but not in melanocytes (pigment-producing cells of the skin).

palliative treatment: treatment that relieves symptoms, such as pain, but is not expected to cure the disease. Its main purpose is to improve the person's quality of life. Sometimes chemotherapy and radiation are used as palliative treatments.

pathologic stage: an estimate of the extent of cancer by direct study of the samples removed during surgery. *See also* clinical stage, molecular staging, staging.

PET scan: *see* positron emission tomography.

positron emission tomography (PET): a PET scan creates an image of the body (or of biochemical events) after the injection of a very low dose of a radioactive form of a substance such as glucose (sugar). The scan computes the rate at which the tumor is using the sugar. In general, high-grade tumors use more sugar than normal and low-grade tumors use less. PET scans are especially useful in taking images of the brain, although they are becoming more widely used to find the spread of cancer of the breast, colon, rectum, ovary, or lung. PET scans may also be used to see how well the tumor is responding to treatment.

prognosis: a prediction of the course of disease; the outlook for the chances of survival.

punch biopsy: *see* biopsy.

quality of life: overall enjoyment of life, which includes a person's sense of well-being and ability to do the things that are important to him or her.

radiation therapy: treatment with high-energy rays (such as x-rays) to kill or shrink cancer cells. The radiation may come from outside of the body (external radiation) or from radioactive materials placed directly in the tumor (brachytherapy or internal radiation). Radiation therapy may be used as the main treatment for a cancer, to reduce the size of a cancer before surgery, or to destroy any remaining cancer cells after surgery. In advanced cancer cases, it may also be used as palliative treatment. *See also* external beam radiation therapy, palliative treatment.

recurrence: the return of cancer after treatment. **Local recurrence** means that the cancer has come back at the same place as the original cancer. **Regional recurrence** means that the cancer has come back after treatment in the lymph nodes near the primary site. **Distant recurrence**, also known as metastatic recurrence, is when cancer metastasizes after treatment to distant organs or tissues (such as the lungs, liver, bone marrow, or brain). *See also* metastasis, metastasize, metastatic.

regional metastasis: *see* metastasis.

reverse transcription polymerase chain reaction (RT-PCR): a highly sensitive laboratory technique for amplifying a defined piece of a ribonucleic acid (RNA) molecule.

risk factor: anything that affects a person's chance of getting a disease such as cancer. Different cancers have different risk factors. For example, unprotected exposure to strong sunlight is a risk factor for skin cancer; smoking is a risk factor for lung, mouth, larynx, and other cancers. Some risk factors, such as smoking, can be controlled. Others, like a person's age, cannot be changed.

seborrheic keratoses: benign raised growths on the skin, usually brown, black or pale and often appearing on the face, chest, shoulders or back. The growth has a waxy, scaly, slightly elevated appearance. Occasionally, a single growth appears, but multiple growths are more common. Typically, seborrheic keratoses do not become cancerous, but they can look like skin cancer. Seborrheic keratoses are common noncancerous (benign) skin growths in older adults.

sentinel lymph node biopsy: a diagnostic procedure involving the removal of the first lymph node to which cancer cells are likely to spread from the primary tumor. In some cases, there can be more than one sentinel lymph node. For this procedure, a radioactive substance or contrast dye is injected near the tumor. A scanner is then used to map the circulation of the substance through the sentinel node. The node is then removed and examined for the presence of cancer cells. *See also* lymph nodes.

shave biopsy: *see* biopsy.

side effects: unwanted effects of treatment, such as hair loss caused by chemotherapy and fatigue caused by radiation therapy.

sign: an observable physical change caused by an illness. *Compare with* symptom.

simple excision: a surgical procedure using a local anesthetic to remove a skin lesion.

skin biopsy: *see* biopsy.

Spitz nevus: a benign, acquired mole derived from melanocytes (pigment cells). This type of nevus generally occurs in children and adolescents, most often on the face and head.

squamous cell: a flat cell that looks like a fish scale under a microscope. These cells are found in the tissues that form the surface of the skin, the lining of the hollow organs of the body (such as the bladder, kidney, and uterus), and the passages of the respiratory and digestive tracts.

squamous cell cancer: *see* squamous cell carcinoma.

squamous cell carcinoma: cancer that begins in squamous cells, which are thin, flat cells that look like fish scales. Squamous cells are found in the tissue that forms the surface of the skin, the lining of the hollow organs of the body, and the passages of the respiratory and digestive tracts.

stage: the extent of a cancer in the body. *See* staging.

staging: the process of finding out whether cancer has spread and, if so, how far. The TNM system, which is used most often, gives 3 key pieces of information:

- T refers to the size of the tumor
- N describes how far the cancer has spread to nearby lymph nodes
- M shows whether the cancer has spread (metastasized) to other organs of the body

Letters or numbers after the T, N, and M give more details about each of these factors. To make this information more clear, the TNM descriptions can be grouped together into a simpler set of stages, labeled with Roman numerals (usually from I to IV). In general, the lower the number, the less the cancer has spread. A higher number means a more serious cancer. *See also* American Joint Committee on Cancer (AJCC) TNM staging system, pathologic stage, clinical stage, molecular staging.

stratum corneum: the outermost layer of the epidermis, which is made up of dead, flat skin cells. The stratum corneum serves as an important barrier, keeping molecules from passing into and out of the skin and thus protecting the lower layers of the skin.

subcutis: the deeper layer of the dermis, containing mostly fat and connective tissue.

sun protection factor (SPF): a number on a scale for rating sunscreens. The SPF rating is calculated by comparing the amount of time needed to produce a sunburn on protected skin to the amount of time needed to cause a sunburn on unprotected skin. Sunscreens with an SPF of 15 or higher are generally thought to provide useful protection from the sun's harmful rays.

symptom: a change in the body caused by an illness, as described by the person experiencing it. *Compare with* sign.

systemic therapy: treatment that reaches and affects cells throughout the entire body, for example, chemotherapy.

tissue: a collection of cells, united to perform a particular function in the body.

TNM staging system: *see* staging.

tumor: an abnormal lump or mass of tissue. Tumors can be benign (noncancerous) or malignant (cancerous).

tumor-infiltrating lymphocyte (TIL): a white blood cell that has left the bloodstream and migrated into a tumor. *See also* lymphocyte.

ulceration: the formation of a break on the skin or on the surface of an organ. An ulcer forms when the surface cells die and are cast off. Ulcers may be associated with cancer and other diseases.

ultraviolet protection factor (UPF): a number on a scale for rating sun-protective clothing for its ability to protect against ultraviolet radiation. The level of protection the garment provides from the sun's UV radiation is rated on a scale from 15 to 50+. The higher the UPF, the higher the protection from UV radiation.

ultraviolet radiation: invisible rays that are part of the energy that comes from the sun. Ultraviolet radiation also comes from sun lamps and tanning beds. It can damage the skin and cause melanoma and other types of skin cancer. Also called UV radiation.

U.S. Food and Drug Administration (FDA): an agency of the United States Department of Health and Human Services. The FDA is responsible for regulating drugs, tobacco products, biological medical products, blood products, medical devices, and radiation-emitting devices, along with other products.

UV Index: a scale ranging from 0 through 11+, used in estimating the risk for sunburn that an unprotected fair-skinned person would have if exposed to the ultraviolet radiation in midday sunlight, accounting for conditions such as cloud cover, ozone, and location.

vaccine: a substance or group of substances meant to cause the immune system to respond to a tumor or to microorganisms, such as bacteria or viruses. A vaccine can help the body recognize and destroy cancer cells or microorganisms.

vitamin D: a nutrient that the body needs in small amounts to function and stay healthy. Vitamin D helps the body use calcium and phosphorus to make strong bones and teeth. It is fat-soluble (can dissolve in fats and oils) and is found in fatty fish, egg yolks, and dairy products. Skin exposed to sunshine can also make vitamin D. Not enough vitamin D can cause a bone disease called rickets. Vitamin D is being studied in the prevention and treatment of some types of cancer. Also called cholecalciferol.

wart: a raised growth on the surface of the skin or other organ.

xeroderma pigmentosum (XP): a genetic condition marked by an extreme sensitivity to ultraviolet radiation, including sunlight. People with xeroderma pigmentosum are not able to repair skin damage from the sun and other sources of ultraviolet radiation and have a very high risk of skin cancer.

x-ray: one form of radiation that can be used at low levels to produce an image of the body on film or at high levels to destroy cancer cells.

Index

Books Published
by the American Cancer Society

Available everywhere books are sold and online at
www.cancer.org/bookstore

Information

*American Cancer Society's Complete Guide to Colorectal
Cancer*

*American Cancer Society Complete Guide to
Complementary & Alternative Cancer Therapies,
Second Edition*

*American Cancer Society Complete Guide to Nutrition for
Cancer Survivors: Eating Well, Staying Well During and
After Cancer, Second Edition*

Breast Cancer Clear & Simple: All Your Questions Answered

QuickFACTS™ - Advanced Cancer

QuickFACTS™ - Basal and Squamous Cell Skin Cancer

QuickFACTS™ - Bone Metastasis

QuickFACTS™ - Breast Cancer

QuickFACTS™ - Colorectal Cancer, Second Edition

QuickFACTS™ - Lung Cancer

QuickFACTS™ - Prostate Cancer, Second Edition

QuickFACTS™ - Thyroid Cancer

Day-to-Day Help

*American Cancer Society Complete Guide to Family
Caregiving, Second Edition*

*American Cancer Society's Guide to Pain Control:
Understanding and Managing Cancer Pain, Revised
Edition*

*Cancer Caregiving A to Z: An At-Home Guide for Patients
and Families*

*Kicking Butts: Quit Smoking and Take Charge of Your
Health, Second Edition*

*Lymphedema: Understanding and Managing Lymphedema
After Cancer Treatment*

What to Eat During Cancer Treatment

When the Focus Is on Care: Palliative Care and Cancer

Emotional Support

*Cancer in the Family: Helping Children Cope with a
Parent's Illness*

Chemo and Me: My Hair Loss Experience

*Couples Confronting Cancer: Keeping Your Relationship
Strong*

*Crossing Divides: A Couple's Story of Cancer, Hope, and
Hiking Montana's Continental Divide*

I Can Survive

*The Survivorship Net: A Parable for the Family, Friends,
and Caregivers of People with Cancer*

*What Helped Get Me Through: Cancer Survivors Share
Wisdom and Hope*

Melanoma

Melanoma is a cancer that begins in the melanocytes. Because most melanoma cells still produce melanin, melanoma tumors are usually brown or black. However, melanomas can also be non-pigmented (no color). They can occur anywhere on the skin, but are more likely to start in certain locations. The trunk (chest and back) is the most common site in men. The legs are the most commonly affected site in women. The neck and face are other common sites for both men and women.

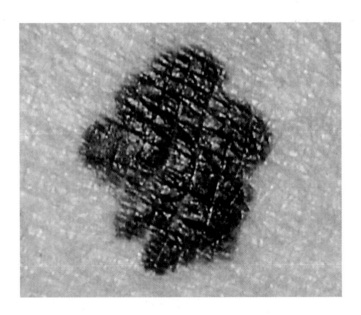

The ABCD rule is a guide to the signs of melanoma:

- **A** is for **Asymmetry:** One half of the mole or birthmark does not match the other.
- **B** is for **Border:** The edges are irregular, ragged, notched, or blurred.
- **C** is for **Color:** The color is not the same all over and may include shades of brown or black or patches of pink, red, white, or blue.
- **D** is for **Diameter:** The spot is larger than 6 mm across (about ¼ inch—the size of a pencil eraser), although melanomas can sometimes be even smaller.

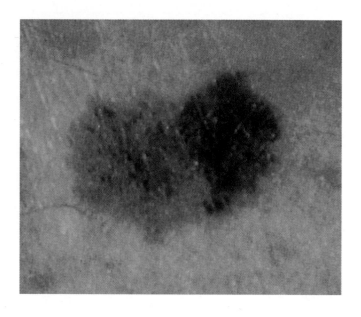

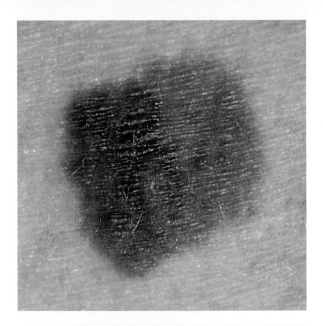

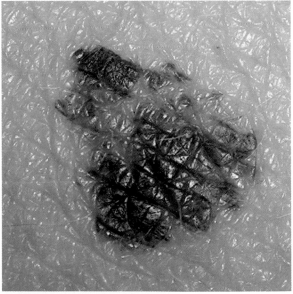

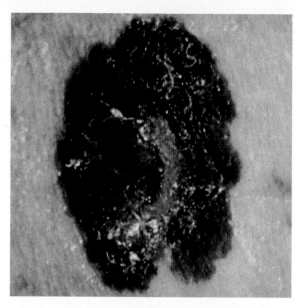

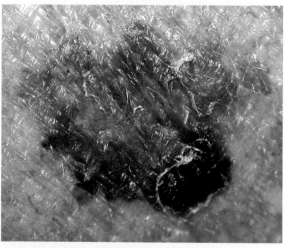

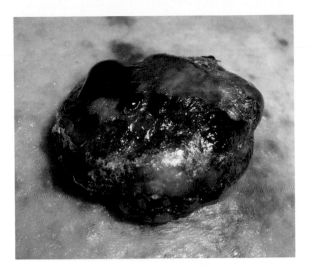

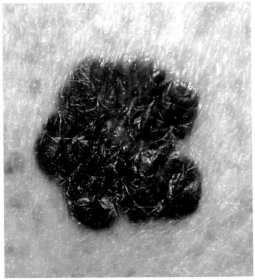

Ways to Reduce Your Risk of Melanoma

1. **Limit Exposure to Ultraviolet Radiation**
   The most important way to lower your risk of melanoma is to protect yourself from exposure to ultraviolet (UV) radiation. Practice sun safety when you are outdoors. Remember this catch phrase: "Slip! Slop! Slap! . . . and Wrap":
   - Slip on a shirt.
   - Slop on sunscreen.
   - Slap on a hat.
   - Wrap on sunglasses to protect the eyes and sensitive skin around them.

2. **Avoid Tanning Beds and Sunlamps**
   Tanning bed use has been linked with an increased risk of melanoma, especially if use is started before the age of 30. Most dermatologists and health organizations recommend not using tanning beds and sunlamps.

3. **Protect Children from the Sun**
   Parents should develop the habit of using sunscreen on exposed skin for themselves and their children whenever they go outdoors and may be exposed to large amounts of sunlight.

4. **Identify Abnormal Moles and Have Them Removed**
   If you have moles, your doctor may want to monitor them with regular examinations or may remove them if their features suggest they could be changing into melanoma.